Copyright © 2016 Mary Lou Shefsky, MPH and Howard A. Pearson, MD. All rights reserved. No part of this book may be reproduced or utilized in any form or by any means, electronic or mechanical, including photocopying, recording, or by information storage and retrieval system, without written permission from the author. Photographs are owned by the individual or organization to whom they are credited along the side of the photo. Photographs without a specific credit are the property of the authors. Photographs may not be reproduced or utilized in any form or by any means without written permission from the owner/photographer.

Designed by Lookbook Press
Seattle, Washington USA

Printed in USA

ISBN: 978-0-692-70437-0 (softbound)

www.fulfillingpaulnewmansdream.org

Facing Page:

The Little Bandit on the left represents the children at The Hole in the Wall Gang Camp. It is from Doc Pearson's 1992 totem pole named FULFILLMENT.

The Little Bandit was originally sketched by graphic artist Andrea Padula at A.E. Hotchner's behest and became Camp's logo, shown on the right. The original bullet hole in the hat was changed to a star in the 1990s.

(Photos courtesy of The Hole in the Wall Gang Camp)

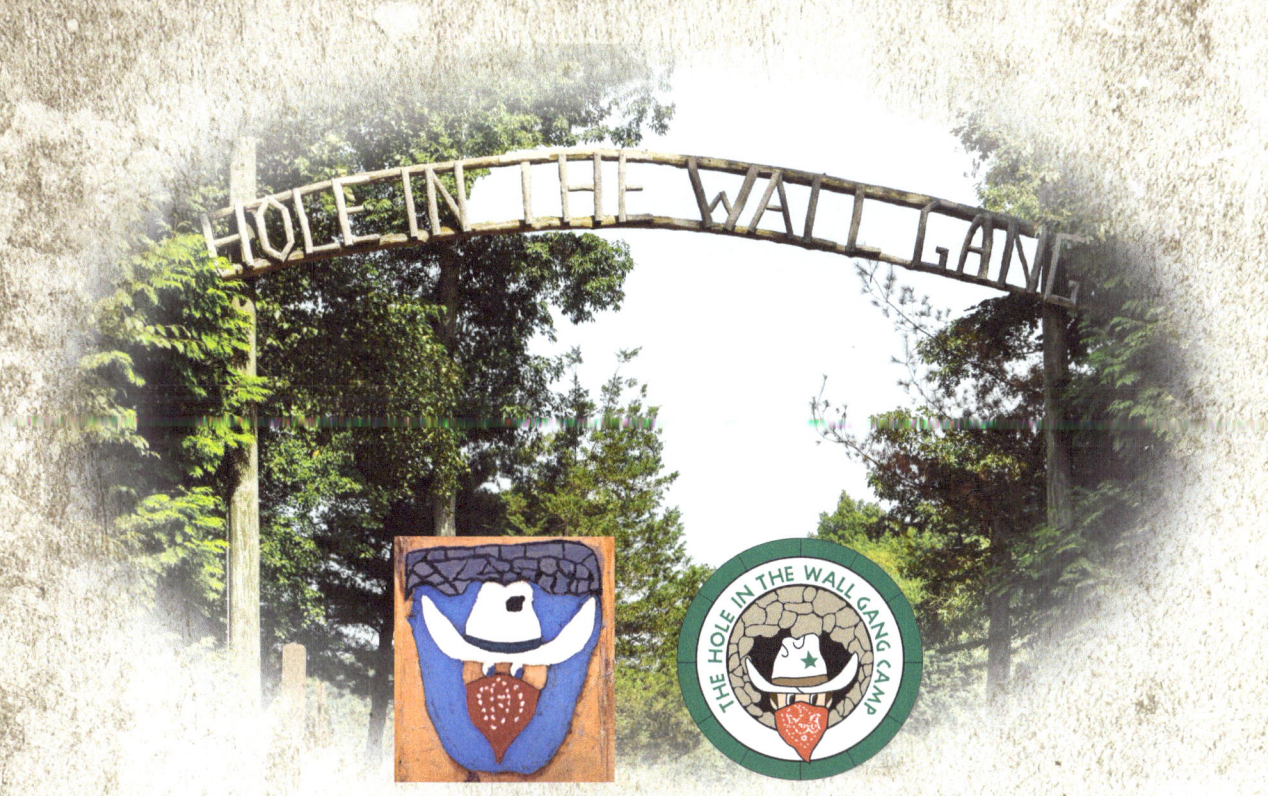

Fulfilling Paul Newman's Dream

"Raising a Little Hell" and Healing at The Hole in the Wall Gang Camp

Howard A. Pearson, MD
Founding Medical Director and "Camp Doc Emeritus"
Mary Lou Shefsky, MPH
Doc's Daughter-in-Law and Camp Volunteer

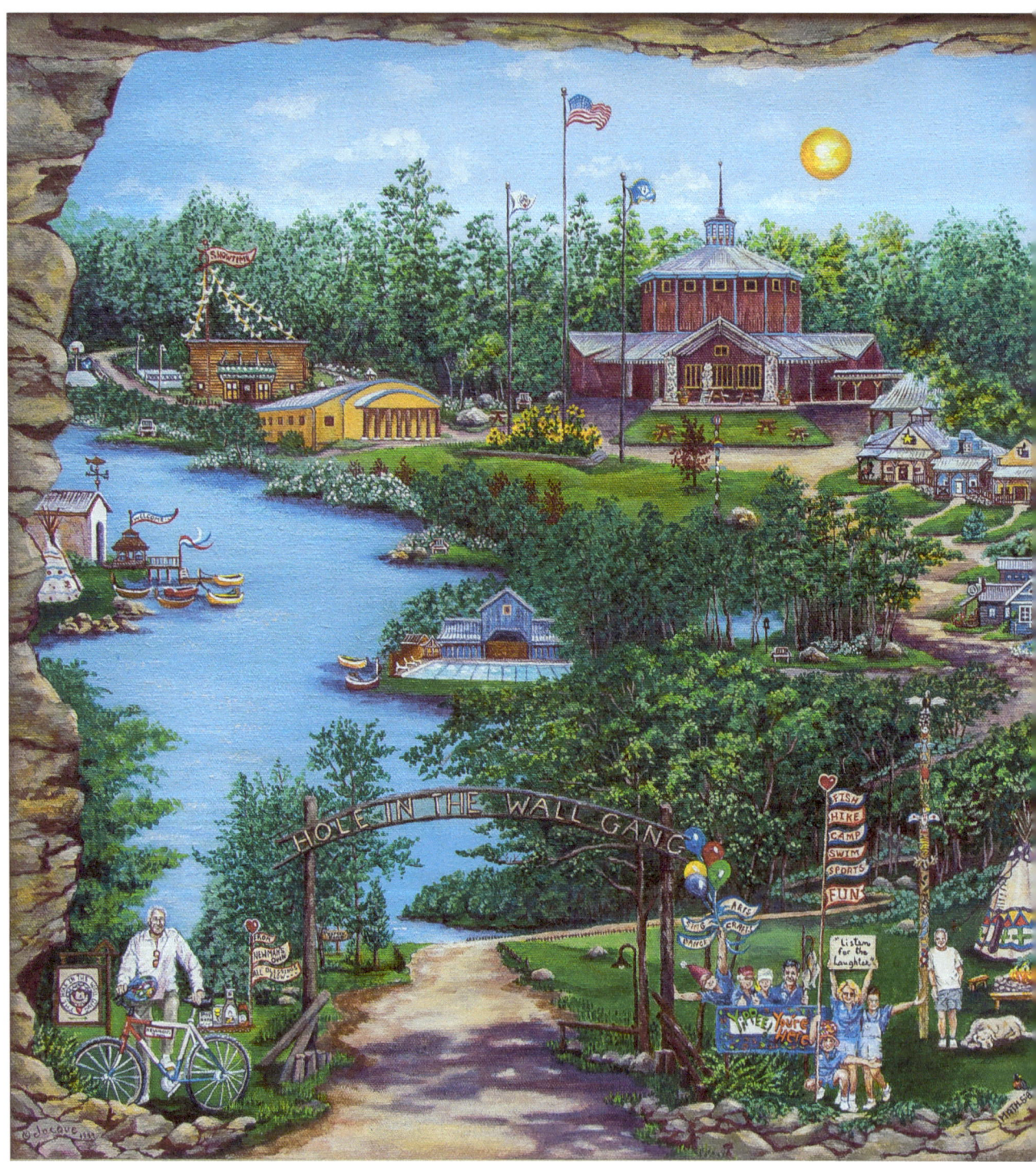

(Photo courtesy of The Hole in the Wall Gang Camp and Jacqué Baker)

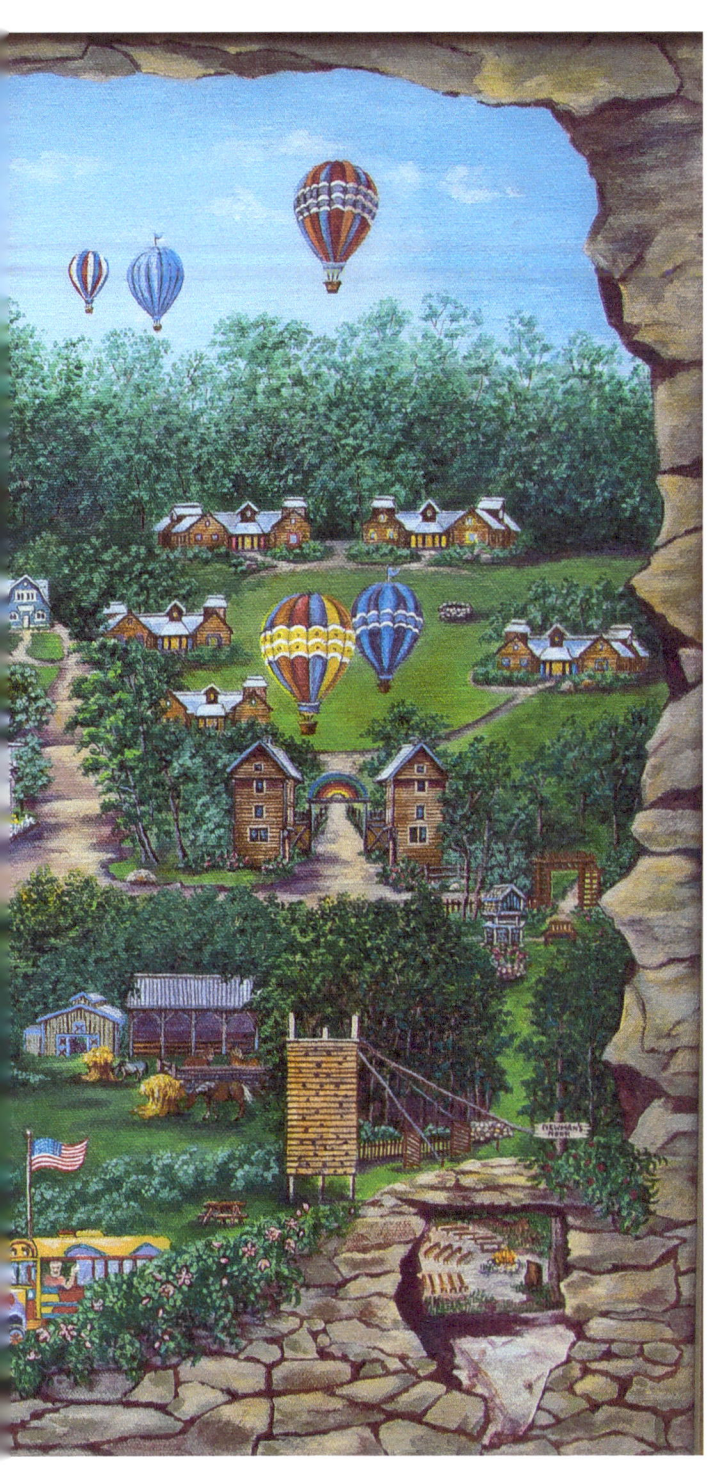

Painting by artist Jacqué Baker, who came to The Hole in the Wall Gang Camp several summers and created this artistic version of it. The painting shows most of the Camp features that are mentioned in this book. Paul Newman is shown in the lower left corner with his decorated bicycle, which he used to get around Camp. Doc Pearson is depicted leaning against his 1992 totem pole called "FULFILLMENT" in the lower center of the painting.

Acknowledgments

First and foremost in acknowledgments is Paul Newman, for his dream and dedicated drive to create The Hole in the Wall Gang Camp (THITWGC or Camp). Without Paul and those who helped to plan and construct the facilities and develop the programs, there would not be Camp nor a book. I extend very special recognition to them and to the campers over the years for their spirit and spunk.

Mary Lou and I drafted the sections pertaining to Camp development and then discussed them with or had them reviewed by Tom Beeby, Vince Conti, Dan Capobianco, Sue Johnson, Bob Wilkins, Dr. Sam Ross, Dr. Nick Evageliou, Dr. Matt Burke, and my granddaughter Jennifer Pearson. In developing the medical sections, we relied heavily upon suggestions from Sue Johnson. Dr. Sharon Space provided data and updates on current medical trends at THITWGC as well as her expert feedback. We also acknowledge Dr. Gary Kupfer, Dr. Eileen Gillan, and Dr. Jack Van Hoff for their review and support. We thank Sue and these four pediatric hematologists/oncologists, all of whom have given a lot of energy and heart to Camp and this book. As we drafted the section on laughter and emotional healing, we had email exchanges and phone conversations with Michael Christensen and some of the Clown Care Unit of the Big Apple Circus--Ilene Weiss, Therese Schorn, Kim Winslow, Maria Peyramaure, and Karen McCarty. Musician Leo Loganov-Katz checked the accuracy of his history. We consulted Dr. Richard Kayne and his daughter Ana on the text that describes their Camp involvement. In 2001, Timothy Hotchner conducted interviews of key people at Camp, which I edited in 2013; they helped affirm my own recollections.

The stunning photographs in the book help convey the spirit and magic of THITWGC. Craig Naumec, Camp's Manager of Media Production, was very helpful in providing photographs from the Archives. Sadly, Craig did not live to see this book published. We give special thanks here for his contribution. We acknowledge THITWGC for permission to independently publish this book and use Archive photographs, which were taken by Craig, Sherry Talley, T. Charlie Erickson, and Mary Harper. We thank Robert Benson for allowing us to use his beautiful photography of the buildings and Bob Sasha for permission to include his *LIFE* magazine 1988 photo of the founders and early supporters of Camp. Artist Jacqué Baker graciously gave us permission to use photos of two of her lovely paintings. My grandson (and Mary Lou's son) Matthew Pearson took a number of the photographs and processed them for this book. His involvement is representative of the family support we both have had during the past several years as we worked on this project. Photographs not showing credits belong to Mary Lou and me.

We asked a number of other people to review successive drafts and make suggestions along the way, including Karen Hendricks (who served on the Board for many years), my son (and Mary Lou's husband) Dr. Stephen Pearson, my grandson (and Mary Lou's son) Daniel Pearson, Dr. Laurie Buchanan, and Mary Lou's cousin Nancy Wishart and friend Dr. Susan Ellis. We acknowledge Camp Chief Executive Officer Jimmy Canton and Board Chairman Ray Lamontagne for their dedication to THITWGC since the beginning as well as for the printing of the totem pole story for internal Camp distribution.

I am grateful for the many friendships that have developed, grown, and endured since the beginning of THITWGC. Friends became my Camp family, and many of them are mentioned in this book. And of course, I appreciate my own family. Mary Lou encouraged me to write this book. Without her co-authorship, it would not have been written. I thank my wife Anne for her loving support for over six decades. She not only painted many of the totems on my poles at Camp, but she also painted seven miniature replicas that I carved. With those miniatures and Mary Lou's cloth replicas in my home, I relive every day many of the wonderful moments at The Hole in the Wall Gang Camp.

Howard A. Pearson, MD
Orange, Connecticut
2016

I wholeheartedly endorse my father-in-law's acknowledgments but would also like to express a few of my own. Having followed my in-laws' involvement with THITWGC beginning in 1986, I am in awe of what was accomplished. I gratefully acknowledge Dad's/Doc's finally relenting to my repeated requests to write about the Camp totem poles ("Doc's Story—The Hole in the Wall Gang Camp and Its Totem Poles") and now "Fulfilling Paul Newman's Dream." I am honored that he allowed me to work with him and that he embraced me as co-author on both of these projects. I treasure the extensive time we have spent writing and editing on the phone between Orange, Connecticut, and Granger, Washington. My husband Stephen has been my main support in many ventures and challenges for over four decades, including this project. Words cannot adequately express my love for and gratitude to him. I thank my son Matthew for his artistic talent and efforts as well as his patience in helping me with technological challenges. I also acknowledge our son Daniel for his constant moral support. A special word of thanks goes to William Hoard of Lookbook Press in Redmond, Washington, for the graphic designing of this book and his enthusiasm.

Stephen, Matthew, Daniel and I spent three sessions in different years at Camp while Dad was Medical Director. While Stephen served as a volunteer pediatrician, I volunteered to fill in wherever I was needed. Because there was space available due to last-minute cancellations, Matthew and Daniel were allowed to stay in the cabins and participate as campers. During our last visit, Matthew was a Leader in Training under the mentorship of Father Dom. Since the early days of planning, we had heard many stories about Camp. We visited it with other Pearson relatives in 1988 after all of the children had left. The physical structures were impressive, but I wondered then how it would feel to be there with the campers and staff. When we finally had the opportunity to participate, The Hole in the Wall Gang Camp came alive for us and changed us for the better.

I have the highest respect for the entire Camp community—the founders, staff, Board, volunteers, campers, and their families—for who they are, what they have done, and what they continue to do with love and courage.

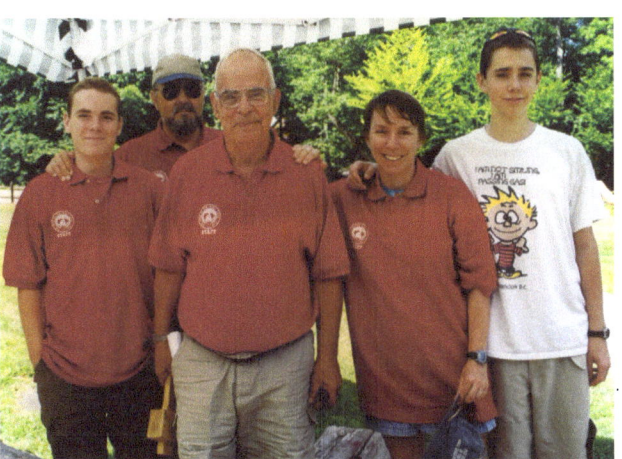

The Pearson-Shefsky Family at Camp in 2001-- From left to right: Matthew, Stephen, Dad/Doc, Mary Lou, and Daniel

Mary Lou Shefsky
Granger, Washington
2016

Preface

"The Hole in the Wall Gang Camp really began with a bottle of salad dressing. It was a sheer accident, as was most everything else we did." - A.E. Hotchner, 2001

The purpose of this book is to share my personal experiences, medical thoughts, and anecdotes about The Hole in the Wall Gang Camp because I think it is an interesting, heart-warming story. With the passing of time, some of these rich memories will be lost unless they are captured in writing. I wrote this book with the help of my daughter-in-law Mary Lou, and we intend to donate any profits from it to Camp.

Physicians and nurses who care for children with life-threatening diseases should find this story worthwhile. Perhaps other people wanting to establish similar camps or programs for children will reflect on what we did to address safety issues and protocols for medical services and back-ups for ill campers. Philanthropists should find this book of interest. Anyone involved in The Hole in the Wall Gang Camp or an affiliate camp—campers, their families, counselors, other staff, and donors—should enjoy reading about how Camp came to be and the first quarter century of its existence from my medical and personal perspective. While this book covers medical aspects and stories from my viewpoint, I encourage others to write in detail about the history of Camp program activities—swimming, horseback riding, boating and fishing, campouts, woodworking and other crafts, and many others—how they developed, how they contribute to the dynamic environment at Camp, and how they help campers heal emotionally.

Based on feedback from children, families, staff, and volunteers, I feel that we have been extraordinarily successful in helping whole families experience emotional healing in the face of coping with life-threatening diseases in children. While A.E. Hotchner might describe most everything we did as "sheer accident," I carefully and thoughtfully planned the medical support at The Hole in the Wall Gang Camp to assure the safety and well being of the children while keeping the medical support non-obtrusive so that the fun aspects of Camp would be possible. Along the way, we all had some amazing experiences. For me personally, it has been one of the most rewarding times of my life.

The Hole in the Wall Gang Camp Board of Directors has given permission to use Camp photographs and independently publish this book. Newman's Own Foundation has approved the use of Paul Newman's name and images in this book. However, their permission is not an endorsement of the book, which is written from my personal perspective.

Howard Pearson

Contents

Dedication	x
Chapter 1 - The Beginning	1
Chapter 2 - Camp Location, Design, and Construction	7
Chapter 3 - Recruiting Campers and Developing the Medical Program	21
Chapter 4 - Additions After Camp's Opening	25
Chapter 5 - Laughter, Music, Dancing, Creativity, and Emotional Healing	31
Chapter 6 - Up and Running	39
Chapter 7 - Celebrities	46
Chapter 8 - Diseases of the Children at Camp	50
Chapter 9 - Special Sessions	62
Chapter 10 - Reflecting on Camp's Past and Looking to the Future	69
Chapter 11 - Beyond Just a Camp Doc	76
Epilogue	107

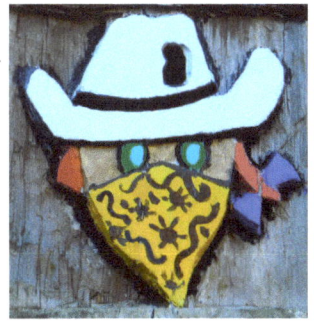

Dedication

This book is dedicated to Paul Newman and his dream
to establish a camp for children with cancer;
to Sue Johnson and Dr. Sharon Space for helping
to make camp medically safe for the children;
and to our campers, whose laughter and joy create
the true magic of The Hole in the Wall Gang Camp.

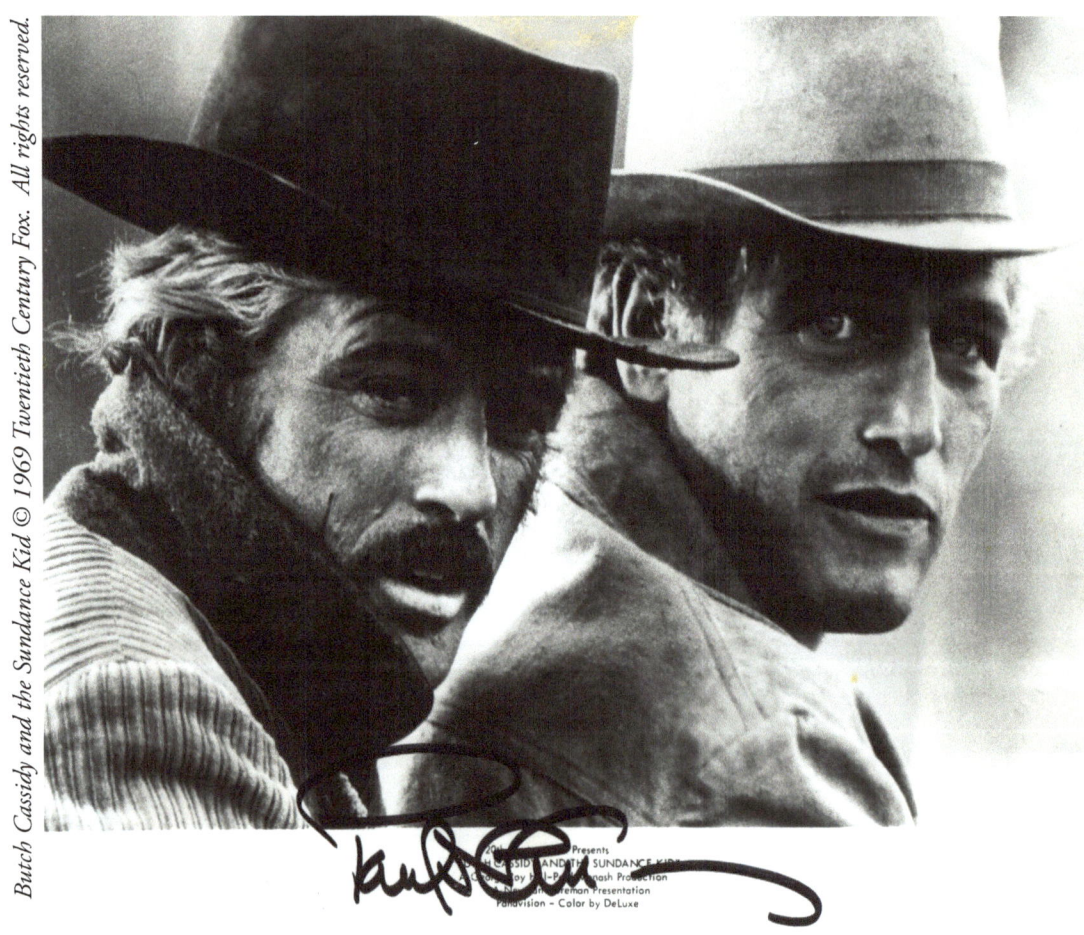

The Stars of *Butch Cassidy and the Sundance Kid*, Robert Redford as the Sundance Kid
on the left and Paul Newman as Butch Cassidy on the right, with Paul's autograph
(Scan of gift to Doc Pearson from Paul Newman)

CHAPTER ONE

The Beginning

"LUCK…How lucky are we who are blessed to have it, and how brutal it is in the lives of unlucky young kids who are struck by serious diseases who don't have time to turn it around."
–Paul Newman, when asked why he wanted to create a summer camp for children with cancer.

The Hole in the Wall Gang Camp (THITWGC or "Camp") was the inspiration and creation of Paul Newman (1925-2008), one of the great American movie actors of the twentieth century. Known for his striking, vivid blue eyes, Paul acted in over 60 motion pictures and directed or produced over ten films. He won numerous awards during his acting career, including an Oscar for Best Actor for his performance in *The Color of Money* (1986), six Golden Globe Awards, and an Emmy Award. Paul was also a professional auto racing driver, team owner, and enthusiast for 35 years. But it was his philanthropy that changed my life and would enrich the lives of thousands of children in New England and subsequently around the world.

In the late 1970's, Paul and his Westport, Connecticut neighbor, author A.E. Hotchner (Hotch) began to distribute bottles of homemade salad dressing to friends at Christmas. The salad dressing was concocted using Paul's recipe and was put in empty wine bottles with an added label that said "Newman's Own." The salad dressing was so well received that in 1981 Paul and Hotch founded Newman's Own food company which, over the next few years, began to produce and sell some food products. This endeavor was very successful. Almost immediately, Newman's Own products were being sold in supermarkets and began to make a profit. They eventually expanded their products to include spaghetti sauce, lemonade, popcorn, cookies, coffee, and other items.

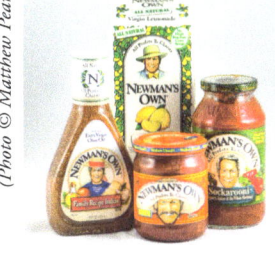

A selection of Newman's Own Products

Because Paul believed that it would be inappropriate for an actor and author to make money from selling food products, he decided that they should annually give all of their profits to selected private, nonprofit 501(c)(3) charities around the country. Under the direction of Paul's Westport attorney Leo Nevas, Newman's Own was set up as a Sub-chapter S corporation that permitted tax-free donations from Newman's Own to charities. After several years, Paul suggested that maybe they should have a charity of their own. They were receiving heartrending letters from parents of desperately ill children, some of whom had cancer. Some families were impoverished by medical expenses, and they asked for money to take their children to Disney World before they died. This was not possible because the tax status of Newman's Own precluded gifts to individuals. Instead, Paul and Hotch decided to create a camp for children with cancer, many of whom would be seriously ill. Attorney Nevas had The Hole in the Wall Gang Camp created as a 501(c)(3) corporation to which tax-deductible money could be given by donors, including Newman's Own.

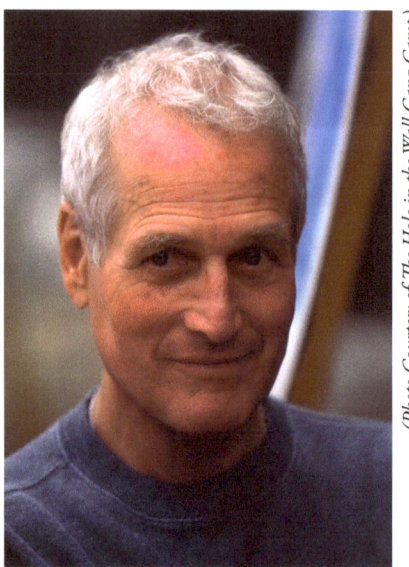

In April 1986, Hotch contacted me and explained Paul Newman's plan to build a camp in Connecticut for children with cancer. I did not know Hotch at the time, but I learned that he was a biographer of Ernest Hemingway and a consultant in movies of Hemingway's books. I knew who Paul Newman was, had seen several of his movies over the years, and was aware that my wife Anne admired his blue eyes.

I knew of summer camp opportunities available for children with specific disease diagnoses, including cancer and sickle cell anemia. These opportunities were made possible by pediatric specialists and community groups working together. Facilities at existing camps were often utilized for part of a summer to host children, sometimes with their families. In 1967, the Sickle Cell Disease Foundation of California created the first summer camp opportunity in the United States for children with sickle cell disease. In 1982, Children's Oncology Camps of America (C.O.C.A.) was founded by 12 existing cancer camp organizations to share ideas, and an international C.O.C.A. was established three years later.[1] To my knowledge, in 1986 there were no existing camps in the United States and perhaps in the world specifically designed from the ground up, constructed, and dedicated to children diagnosed with cancer or life-threatening blood diseases. When Hotch came to my office at Yale-New Haven Hospital that April, we talked for about an hour. He told me that he had met Paul on a movie set in Hollywood. They had been fast friends for more than 35 years and were partners in the Newman's Own food company. The food business was very successful and generated profits which they wanted to donate to their own charity, and they had decided that it would be a camp for children with cancer in Connecticut. I asked why they wanted to build it in Connecticut. Hotch explained that he and Paul lived in Westport, and they wanted the camp to be located near them.

Why had they come to me? In order to create their camp, Paul and Hotch realized that they would need input from a physician, preferably a pediatric hematologist/oncologist, concerning the camper population and the degree of illness that could be accepted and safely managed. They had also decided that the doctor who would be their Medical Director should be from Connecticut. Paul had Yale connections, having attended the Yale School of Drama. Leo Nevas began asking

Blue-eyed Paul, 1990

(Photo Courtesy of The Hole in the Wall Gang Camp)

---

1   http://www.cocai.org/index.php/about-cocai/history-of-cocai

around who might be the right Yale pediatric oncologist to contact. By chance at a cocktail party in Woodbridge, Connecticut, Leo met Dr. Richard Ehrenkranz, one of my Yale colleagues, who suggested my name. I had established the first pediatric hematology/oncology service in Connecticut at Yale in 1968. At the time I met with Hotch, I was the senior pediatric hematologist/oncologist in Connecticut, had been Chairman of the Department of Pediatrics at Yale School of Medicine since 1974, had many years of experience treating children with cancer and blood diseases, and had worked closely with families and community groups. In addition, I had done research on some of these diseases.

At that first meeting, Hotch told me that Paul said that the camp would be called "The Hole in the Wall Gang Camp." The name came from Paul's favorite movie, *Butch Cassidy and the Sundance Kid*, involving a rag tag group of Wild West outlaws called the Hole in the Wall Gang. The movie was based on the lives of real men, with Paul playing the role of Butch Cassidy and Robert Redford portraying the Sundance Kid. Just as the Hole in the Wall Pass in Wyoming served as a refuge and hideout in the movie, the camp envisioned by Paul would be a specially designed refuge and hideout where children could "raise a little hell" and have fun among supportive peers and counselors. Also, Paul wanted it "built yesterday!" I asked Hotch why Paul wanted to develop a camp for children with cancer. He replied that although Paul did not have family or close friends who had a child with cancer, he had once said that the thing that motivated him most was "LUCK—How lucky are we who are blessed to have it, and how brutal it is in the lives of unlucky young kids who are struck by serious diseases who don't have time to turn it around."

A few weeks later, I met Paul for the first time. He invited my wife Anne and me to dinner at a very nice restaurant in Westport to talk about his ideas for a camp. I learned that he had visited cancer camps in California and New Jersey where he had been told that having strong medical involvement was essential. At dinner, Paul's youngest daughter, Clea, accompanied him. As a pediatrician, I always observe how parents interact with their children and vice versa. It was evident that Paul and Clea adored each other. I was impressed with this aspect of Paul's character. Afterwards, Anne was the envy of some of her friends when she told them she had met Paul Newman and his eyes were strikingly blue!

After the dinner, I realized that, given the size of the camp being considered, it would have the capacity to serve about 800 children each summer. I knew it could not be only for Connecticut children. In the entire United States, only about 15,800 children from birth to 19 years of age are diagnosed with cancer annually.[2] Even if campers were drawn from all of New England, I was dubious that we could fill to capacity each summer. I knew that we would need to expand the mission. Without much arm-twisting, I convinced Paul that the mission should also include children with serious blood diseases such as sickle cell anemia, thalassemia major, and hemophilia. These children are cared for by the same physicians who treat children with cancer. While internal medicine has separate sub-boards, one in oncology and another in hematology, pediatrics has a single sub-board that covers both specialties. Also, virtually all children with these conditions are cared for in clinics affiliated with medical schools because there are very few pediatric hematologist/oncologists in private practice.

A short time later, Hotch and Paul asked me to become the first Medical Director of The

---

2   Childhood Cancers, National Cancer Institute Fact Sheet, 2014 <http://www.cancer.gov/cancertopics/factsheet/Sites-Types/childhood>.

Hole in the Wall Gang Camp. At the time, I was stepping down as Chairman of Pediatrics at Yale after serving in the position for 12 years. I thought that I would have some free time. I initially believed that I would be a consultant and merely give advice about recruiting campers, deciding how sick they could be, addressing issues about the medical and nursing staff, planning the medical and nursing procedures, and providing medical backup.

Paul attracted a talented group of individuals who constituted Camp's first Board of Directors. Hotch was an obvious selection, given his partnership in the food company and early involvement with the camp idea. His wife Ursula was included for her energy and interest in the project. Attorney Leo Nevas joined the Board for his legal expertise. Ray Lamontagne became a member because of his experience in raising money for charitable causes. Ray, a Yale University undergraduate and law school graduate who had helped Sargent Shriver set up the Peace Corps program in the early 1960s, had worked with the Rockefeller Foundation as a fund-raiser. Dr. Samuel (Sam) Ross, founder of Green Chimneys Children's Services,[3] willingly served on the Board. Sam was especially motivated because he had a son who died of Hodgkin's disease, cancer of the lymph glands. Simon Konover, head of a large construction firm in Hartford (the Simon Konover Company), was hired as the building contractor for Camp and became a Board member.

I was successful in recruiting Vincent (Vince) Conti as a Board member. Vince was a Vice President at Yale-New Haven Hospital from 1978 until 1997, when he became Chief Executive of Maine Medical Center in Portland. His special assignment at Yale was pediatrics. As Chairman of Pediatrics, I had worked with him closely in planning the new Yale-New Haven Children's Hospital and was impressed by his mastery of regulations that pertained to the care of children. I knew that the original Board would require someone with regulatory expertise. Vince's guidance was crucial in the founding of Camp.

Including Paul, Hotch, and me, we had a Board of nine. The Board met frequently in 1986 and 1987 to review plans and resolve issues related to THITWGC. By the time the property was purchased in September 1986, there already had been many discussions about the children we would serve. Paul's presence and leadership dominated the direction of the meetings and influenced the scope, design, and style of Camp.

Based on initial architectural plans, land purchase, and construction, the first estimate of the project's cost was $8,000,000. Newman's Own could donate half of this amount, but the other half had to come from donations from other sources in order to comply with non-profit regulations. Simon Konover soon revised the estimate to $12,000,000. The effort to raise matching funds was headed by Ray Lamontagne, who was helped by Shivaun Manley at the Newman's Own office. A number of significant gifts were obtained, including one from Anheuser Bush (a sponsor of Paul's racing cars) that paid for the Dining Hall and one from the Dyson Foundation that paid for the Infirmary. But the most spectacular gift came from the Kingdom of Saudi Arabia.

Ray had mentioned Paul's plan for THITWGC to a close friend in Washington, D.C., and had sent him some information about it. In turn, this friend shared the information with a young Saudi Arabian man named Khaled Alhegelan who told him, "I have thalassemia major, a serious blood disease that requires blood transfusions every month. I would have loved to go to a camp

---

[3] Green Chimneys is a multi-faceted nonprofit organization based in Brewster, New York that provides residential, clinical, recreational, and educational services to at-risk young people. It was a pioneer in animal-assisted therapy (AAT). See http://www.greenchimneys.org.

like this, but I never had the chance. It sounds terrific. I'd like to talk to Paul Newman about it." Ray arranged a time for Khaled to visit the Newman's Own office to meet Paul. At the time, the office had only a ping-pong table and lawn chairs as furniture. After talking with Paul about the camp, Khaled challenged him to a game of ping-pong. Before they started, Khaled commented, "I bet you're going to let me win." Paul responded, "Hell, no!" and proceeded to beat him soundly.

Before leaving, Khaled mentioned that Saudi citizens could petition their King for gifts and that he would make a request on behalf of Camp. Amongst ourselves, there was speculation that we might receive $10,000 to $50,000. Two or three weeks later, I received a call from Paul who asked whether I thought the medical establishment of Connecticut would be upset if Camp accepted a gift from Saudi Arabia. I asked if there were any strings attached. He said that there were two: 1) He (Paul) had to personally attend a press conference in Washington, D.C., and 2) The check had to be presented at a reception the same evening at the Saudi Arabian Embassy. I did not think anyone would be upset and urged Paul to agree. There had actually been a third stipulation—Khaled had wanted to personally tell Paul about the generous gift, which Ray had easily arranged.

Khaled had approached the Saudi Ambassador to the United States, Prince Bandar, who

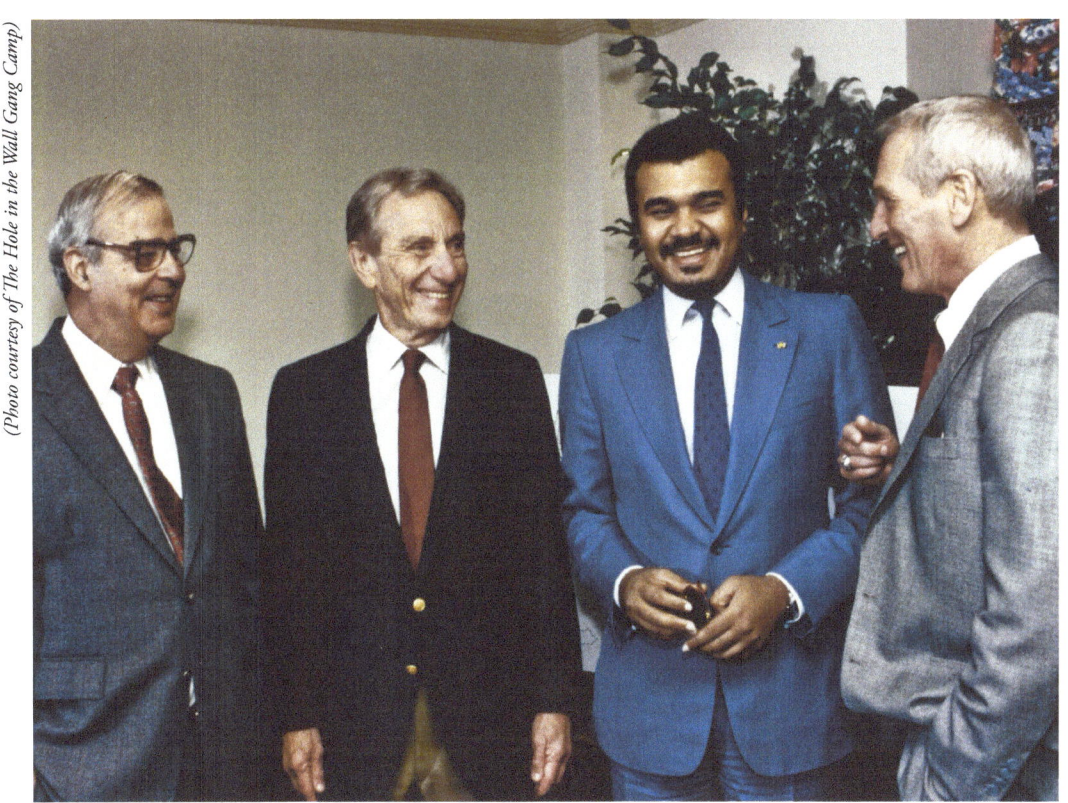

(Photo courtesy of The Hole in the Wall Gang Camp)

Reception at the Saudi Arabian Embassy,
Left to right: Doc, Hotch, Prince Bandar, and Paul

then spoke with His Majesty, King Fahad. This resulted in the presentation of a $5,000,000 check to Paul by Prince Bandar at a lavish but non-alcoholic reception. This gift from the King was on behalf of the Saudi people. Although the Saudis asked for nothing else, Shivaun Manley in the Newman's Own office had an appreciatory plaque placed on a large boulder at Camp acknowledging the gift. Khaled later became an active member of the Camp Board of Directors; he is still a Board member in 2016. With the contribution by Newman's Own and other gifts, a total of $20,000,000 was raised that covered the costs of site purchase and construction as well as the establishment of a significant endowment.

Ray has commented that fundraising for Camp turned out to be relatively easy, in large part because it was a venture devised and led by Paul Newman. Ray had first met Paul at a gathering of Connecticut businessmen in an attempt to begin raising money from sources outside of Newman's Own. The gathering was held in Paul's barn, an elegantly remodeled structure for entertaining behind his home in Westport where he displayed family memorabilia, including the Oscar awarded for Best Actress to his wife, Joanne Woodward, for her role in *The Three Faces of Eve* (1958). In attendance was the Governor of Connecticut, William O'Neill, who was an early supporter of the venture and who had provided Paul with a list of businessmen to invite. At that event and other fund-raisers, potential donors were interested in meeting the movie star. For the sake of making Camp happen, Paul often met with potential donors but always wanted the focus to be on Camp rather than on him.

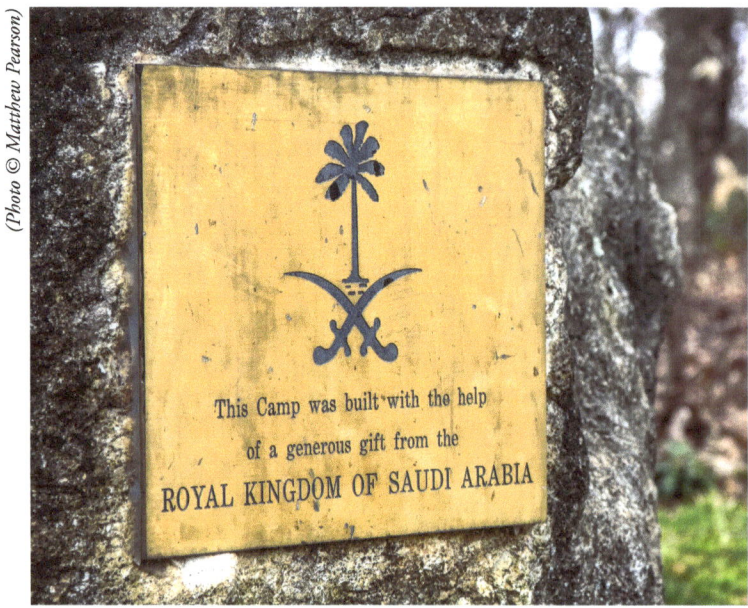

Boulder with Saudi plaque

CHAPTER TWO

Camp Location, Design, and Construction

"Paul's theory of architecture was that whenever you had to decide to design buildings that were either more the same or more different, always make them more different." – Tom Beeby

Paul had some clear ideas about Camp, beyond the fact that it would be in Connecticut. He wanted the site to be large, heavily forested, a distance from busy highways to assure privacy and safety, have a large lake, and have topography that could be made accessible for children with mobility problems. He insisted that the facilities would not look institutional or hospital-like and would have the flavor of an old western town. The spring and summer of 1986 were spent looking at possible sites.

A facility for handicapped children that was not used in the summer was offered but was not considered because it appeared too institutional for Paul's liking. Paul assessed a regional water company property near New Haven by flying over it in a helicopter but rejected it because it was too small, too close to the city, and had a high voltage power line running through it. An abandoned Boy Scout camp owned by the YMCA in Torrington was offered, but the YMCA said that the property and lake would have to be shared with the Boy Scouts. In addition, the terrain was too hilly for children with handicaps.

A property on the Connecticut River outside of Old Lyme was on the market and brought to our attention. Because this property was near the epicenter of a Lyme disease epidemic, I vetoed it. In the early 1970s, a child from the area was referred to the rheumatology clinic at Yale with a swollen, painful knee and was diagnosed as having rheumatoid arthritis. When the mother was told of this diagnosis, she commented, "That's strange, because three other children on my street have been given this diagnosis." Doctors Allen Steere and Stephen Malawista at the Yale School of Medicine investigated this further. They found clusters of this diagnosis in three contiguous eastern Connecticut communities, including Lyme and Old Lyme. They published their results in 1977,[1] naming the condition "Lyme disease." It was determined to be a tick-borne bacterial disease

---

1   AC Steere, et al., "Lyme arthritis: an epidemic of oligoarticular arthritis in children and adults in three Connecticut communities," *Arthritis Rheum*. Jan-Feb:20(1), (1977): 7-17.

CHAPTER 2 ~ Camp Location, Design, and Construction

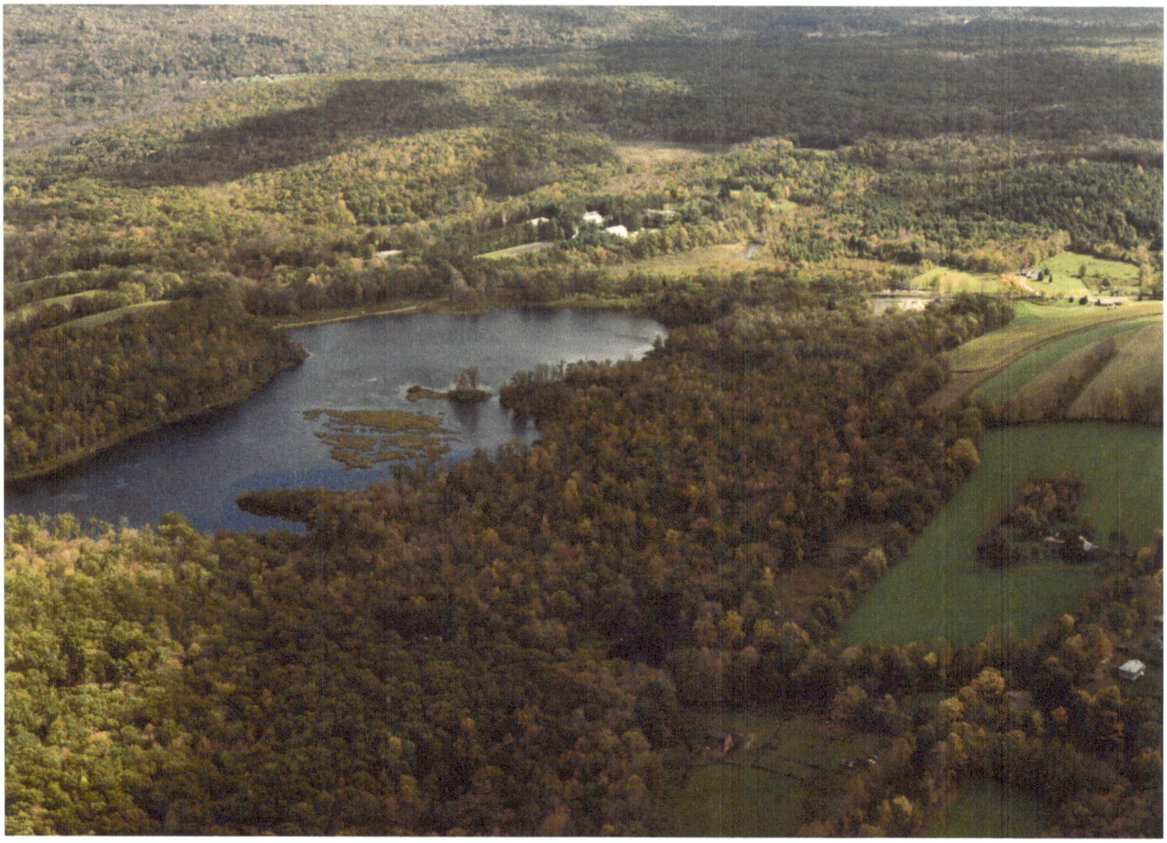

Aerial view of the property before Camp, 1986

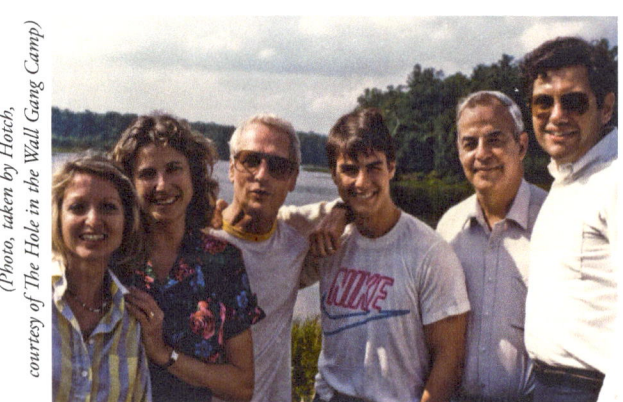

*At the first site visit in July 1986 to what became Camp.
Left to right: Ursula, Mimi Rogers, Paul,
Tom Cruise, Doc, and Vince Conti*

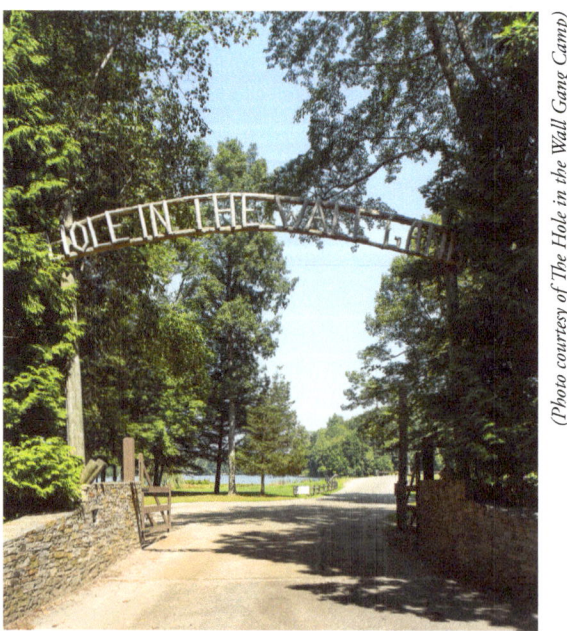

Entrance to Camp

that can initially cause fever, a unique bull's-eye rash, headache, and fatigue. If not diagnosed and treated, problems in the joints (thus the rheumatoid arthritis consideration), heart, and central nervous system can occur.[2] I did not know what Lyme disease might do to immuno-compromised children, and I did not want to find out!

In July 1986, Vince Conti and I were included in a visit to a property on the market in the towns of Ashford and Eastford in northeastern Connecticut. He and I were asked to meet Paul at the exit by the last tollbooth on the Wilbur Cross Parkway. Vince and I thought we would drive with him from that point and get some perspective of how a real race car driver drives. But because there was no room in Paul's car (Hotch was the front passenger and a man and a woman were in the backseat), we followed Paul for 70 miles to the property. When we stopped for lunch in Ashford, one of the backseat occupants from Paul's car introduced himself as Tom Cruise and called me "sir." At the time, Paul and Tom were filming *The Color of Money*, which would win Paul an Academy Award for Best Actor. I had no clue as to Tom's celebrity until after the visit, when I asked my granddaughter Jennifer who Tom Cruise was, and she shrieked and nearly fainted.

A couple of years later, I personally had the opportunity to ride to Camp with Paul the race car driver. While on Interstate 84, we heard a siren and saw flashing red lights behind us. Paul pulled to the side of the highway and stopped. A State trooper approached the car and sternly asked, "Do you realize you were speeding?" Then he stared at Paul and inquired with awe, "Are you Paul Newman?" When Paul nodded his head, the trooper directed him to, "Get back on the road and get out of here! If I gave you a ticket, my wife would kill me!"

The Ashford/Eastford property was a heavily forested 300-acre tract with a 45-acre man-made lake that owner Stephen Harakaly and his sons had created by building a dam across a stream. This definitely met one of Paul's criteria of a lake or large pond that would be used for boating, fishing, and swimming. While we were hiking around the property during this first visit, Paul was plagued by clouds of black flies and mosquitoes buzzing around him. In an attempt to repel them, he collected and put some fern fronds on his head. Although it did not seem to help much, Paul made all of us laugh. From the first moments, we felt relaxed on this property.

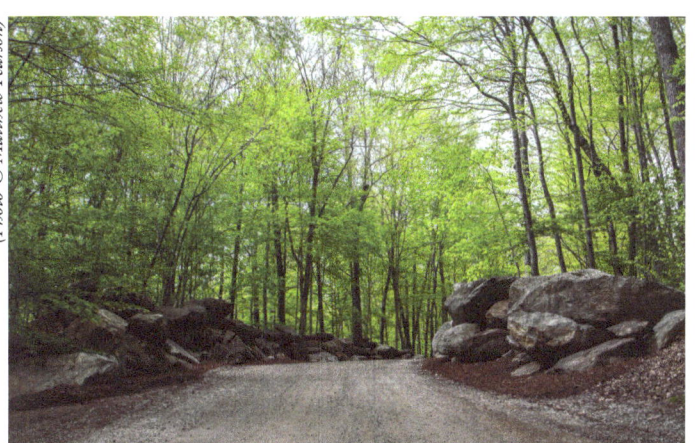

Boulders lining the road into Camp

(Photo © Matthew Pearson)

There were only a few narrow paths through the woods and no buildings or utilities. Several cleared areas at the back of the property where Camp buildings could be constructed were far from a busy highway. The topography had no high hills and could be graded to assure accessibility. Ashford-Eastford is 33 miles from Hartford, 68 from New Haven, 40 from Providence, 82 from Boston, and 145 miles from New York City. This parcel of land seemed to meet all of Paul's criteria. It also met mine—centrally located in order to draw children from throughout New England and

---

2   http://en.wikipedia.org/wiki/Lyme_disease

adaptability for children with mobility issues.

All of us felt that we had found the site for THITWGC. Subsequent visits by Paul and others were reinforcing, in spite of Paul's continued problem with black flies and mosquitoes. I heard that he was more successful in repelling them by donning a white chef's hat smeared with jam. Even more than 25 years later, the property still provides the sense of a secluded refuge for children that Paul originally envisioned. Starting with the entrance to the property off of Route 44, children come into this special place by passing under a rustic arch of tree branches forming the name of THITWGC, proceeding on the road built on top of the dam, and then going on a stretch of road lined on each side by enormous boulders representing the wall that children are passing through to their safe place.

The Ashford-Eastford property was purchased at a press conference at Yale-New Haven Hospital in September 1986 from Stephen Harakaly. His son George, who had grown up on the property and still lived directly adjacent it, became the first Maintenance Director. Like his father and brothers, George was a skillful carpenter and knew how to fix things. He was well respected in Ashford, which helped promote a good Camp-town relationship. A formal groundbreaking ceremony of The Hole in the Wall Gang Camp was held in Ashford on December 6, 1986. Governor William O'Neill, Senator Joseph Lieberman, and many news reporters attended it. Paul formally announced that Camp would open in June 1988, only 18 months down the line.

Everyone but Paul felt that it would be impossible to design and build a functional camp of the projected size and complexity in such a short time. I have said many times that if this had been a Yale Medical School or Yale-New Haven Hospital project, we would probably have done feasibility studies for several years! If there were any possibility of meeting Paul's deadline, planning would need to begin promptly.

We had to find an architect as soon as possible. I called Thomas H. Beeby (Tom), who was the Dean of the Yale School of Architecture as well as the Chairman of Hammond, Beeby, Rupert, Ainge (HBRA), a large and prestigious architectural firm based in Chicago. I asked Tom whether he knew of any architects specializing in the design of camps that we could contact. He said he did not but asked me why I wanted to know. When I told him about Paul's plans, he offered to become involved. Tom and his firm agreed to plan Camp's layout and design its buildings, which they did over the next nine months. They only billed for minimal managerial costs.

Active planning of the layout and the design of the buildings began in earnest in the spring and summer of 1987. Tom and Tannys Langdon, a member of his firm,

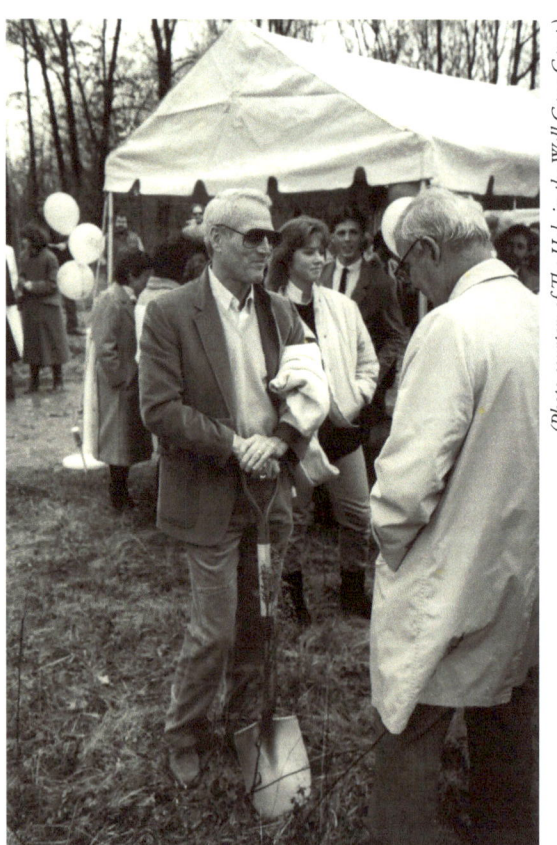

At the groundbreaking, with Paul. My granddaughter Jennifer and son Douglas are in the background

(Photo courtesy of The Hole in the Wall Gang Camp)

made preliminary drawings of the buildings, which were then reviewed by Paul, who continued to insist that Camp would not be institutional or hospital-like, but would have a western flavor. Camp obviously had to have a medical aspect, but it should not be conspicuous. Tom came up with the idea of making the layout look like a rural town with a green surrounded by public buildings. These buildings were separated from a residential circle of cabins by a gate between two buildings with the appearance of a fort or stockade. The residential circle was divided into five Units, each assigned a distinct color (blue, red, yellow, green, and white), and three cabins. (In 1989, white was changed to purple when it was realized during the first Sickle Cell Session, explained later, that there were racial implications pertaining to the Unit color. When the Unit leader called out to the African-American campers, "All you White guys, assemble for lunch," there was no response. I mention this as a caution to camp developers in the future to carefully think about these kinds of details.)

Since we would have campers between seven and 15 years of age and of both genders, the Unit design provided for flexibility. While originally the cabin design accommodated six campers and three counselors, we later increased the camper capacity to 10 or 12 per cabin by including bunk beds and the counselor capacity to four to provide adequate support for the children. This cabin ratio, along with activity volunteers, contributes greatly to making Camp a safe medical environment that is emotionally supportive for campers. In other summer camps and in public school settings these days, hugging of children is discouraged. However, at Camp it is encouraged and practiced because comforting physical contact is part of the emotional healing of our children.

Tom also convinced Paul that the buildings themselves did not have to be specifically western. While log cabins could be used for the residential circle, farm structures or lumber mills could be models for the public buildings. When I asked Tom what his overriding design theme of Camp buildings was, he replied, "They are a collage of American architectural genres." The Administration building resembles a village town hall, while the Infirmary has the look of an Oregon sawmill. The Arts & Crafts building is similar to shops on a block of a village road. A Shaker barn was the inspiration for the massive, dark red circular Dining Hall with its towering roof topped by a cricket weather vane. The Gymnasium has the exterior look of an Oregon bow barn. I have often said that THITWGC is the "Taj Mahal" of summer camps! In 1993, Tom's design received the American Institute of Architects' most distinguished recognition, a National Honor Award.

After Paul approved a preliminary drawing of a building, one of the HBRA architects was assigned to develop specific, detailed plans. Each architect was given the preliminary drawing as well as guidelines to determine the size and location of the building. This process of design insured a maximum variety of structures and allowed multiple buildings to be developed simultaneously. The architect would then make a detailed construction design, bring it to Connecticut, and present it to the Board for final approval. Discussion was candid, and everyone freely offered opinions. Board member Dr. Sam Ross so frequently asked, "Where are the toilets? We need more!" that we called him the "Toilet Man." We were thoughtful and proactive in our planning but occasionally had to make adjustments when a shortcoming was brought to our attention.

In addition to planning and constructing over 35 buildings, infrastructure had to be installed, including a water system, septic tanks, telephone lines, an underground electrical network, roads, and pathways. Everything had to be planned and built with handicapped access.

By September 1987, little had been done on the site except for cutting down some trees where the roads were planned. There were no buildings under construction and no infrastructure in place. A number of permits had to be obtained from the local town officials. When Tom met with them in the back room of the Ashford library to present the preliminary site plans, they raised roadblocks and were not very helpful. A second meeting, held by Tom a month later in the school gymnasium, was attended by Paul, Leo Nevas, Vince Conti, and me, as well as 400 townspeople! Leo and Vince assured the town fire marshal that the property and buildings would not function as a health facility but rather as a camp, and that there were different requirements and codes than those needed for hospitals or health care facilities. I assured them that Camp would pose no health hazards to the towns. By the end of the meeting, there was consensus that anything Paul wanted was fine.

At some early point, town officials of Ashford and Eastford expressed concerns that their small communities would lose revenue because of Camp's non-profit status, which made it exempt from property taxes. Paul and Vince, guided by Leo, attended town meetings to address their concerns and defuse the issue. The towns were promised that THITWGC would annually donate the amount collected from property taxes as they were assessed to them in 1986. The towns were also assured that there would be no full-time employees living on the property year-round whose children might need to be enrolled in local schools. Paul's earnestness in addressing their concerns promoted good local relationships that allowed development at a super-rapid pace.

Simon Konover assigned a young man, Michael (Mike) Kolakowski, as the on-site Project Director. When Simon introduced Mike to Paul, he was taken aback by Mike's youthful appearance. Paul pulled Simon aside and asked him, "Why are you sending a private to do a general's job?" Simon replied, "He's a general. Just wait and see." Simon obviously had a lot of confidence in Mike, and the Project Director eventually exceeded everyone's expectations.

Construction began in earnest in the winter of 1987 and continued through the spring of 1988, often occurring seven days a week. All needed utilities were installed. Local well diggers dug four deep wells for free to provide all the water that Camp would need. The contour of the land was shaped to eliminate steep slopes that could impede wheelchairs or crutches. Golf carts would be available to take campers to the outlying areas such as the Boat House and the camp-out

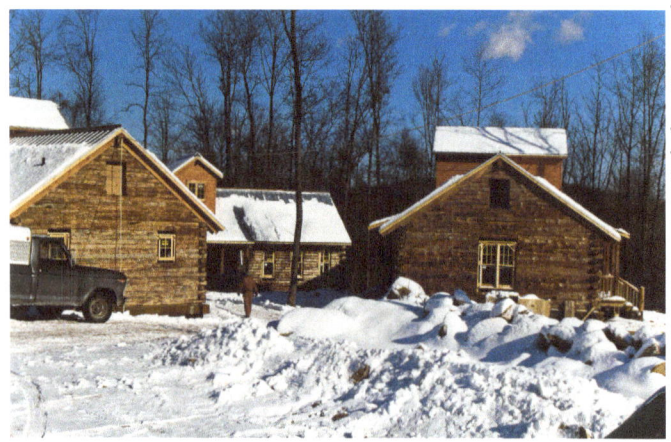

Cabins built during the harsh winter

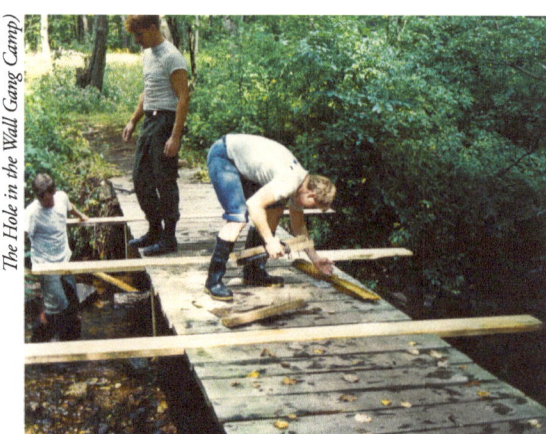

Navy Seabees building a bridge

(Both photos Courtesy of The Hole in the Wall Gang Camp)

area, where children enjoy activities around campfires and tepees. While accessibility was essential, obvious ramps and stairs were kept to a minimum. All of the buildings were designed so that they would be accessible from the ground level. This was so skillfully done that handicapped accessibility is not noticeable unless someone is looking for it. Whenever there was a delay in obtaining State permits, Paul called the Governor and they would be issued the next day!

Construction was hampered by harsh winter weather with snow and mud on the roads. Paul had insisted that the roads would not be paved because he wanted an "Old West" atmosphere. However, work moved so swiftly that construction of a building was often begun before the final plans for it were completed. Fifteen log cabins, divided into a ring of five Units, were built in the winter by a Canadian crew used to working in the cold.

The Connecticut U.S. Navy Reserve Construction Battalion (often called CBs or Seabees) built paths and bridges through the site's wetlands during their two weeks of active duty that spring. The Seabees also cleared an area on the edge of the pond for a beach, with the intent that the children would swim in the pond. However, in the process, the Seabees encountered large non-venomous water snakes, prompting the rethinking of how to provide campers an enjoyable swimming experience. I mention this not to alarm people but rather to urge vigilance and thoughtfulness. The presence of potentially harmful or upsetting fauna and flora in the environment (including reptiles, mosquitoes, ticks, and poison ivy) should be taken into consideration during the planning, development, and service delivery at any summer camp but particularly one serving children with life-threatening diseases.

As a result of the snake discovery, a swimming pool company was contacted. The owner was very excited about helping and wanted to donate the labor but would have to get other pool companies to participate due to the size of the project. He organized a group of Connecticut swimming pool contractors who temporarily put aside their usual cutthroat competitiveness and jointly designed and built *pro bono* an Olympic-size heated swimming pool. The pool met my specifications for safety—the maximum depth was five feet and there were no diving boards. One contractor dug the hole, another put the cement in, another laid the tiles, one did the plumbing, and yet another constructed the dressing rooms. When the swimming facilities were completed, the contractors had a celebration, which included blessings of the pool and Camp by a Catholic priest, Protestant minister, and Jewish rabbi. Paul reflected, "A sense of community was present with almost everything that was done at Camp."

In addition to planning for arts & crafts, a camp-out area, and other traditional summer camp activities, Dr. Sam Ross felt strongly about the calming effect that domesticated animals can have on people in general and children in particular. He advocated including a Horse Barn with riding opportunities for campers. This provided me with the medical challenge of planning for all campers to ride safely. From the beginning, the Horse Barn was a popular activity. THITWGC was the first summer camp in New England and one of the very earliest in the country to allow boys with hemophilia, a genetic condition that puts them at risk of bleeding, to ride horses. Two camps affiliated with the National Hemophilia Foundation preceded us.[3] It is important for the safety of boys with hemophilia to have medical supervision and treatment capabilities on site.

---

3   The Mile High Camp in Colorado began this activity in 1979, and Camp Ailihpomeh (hemophilia spelled backward) in Texas has provided it since at least 1986. None of the other camps responding to our inquiries offered horseback riding earlier than 1988.

CHAPTER 2 ~ Camp Location, Design, and Construction

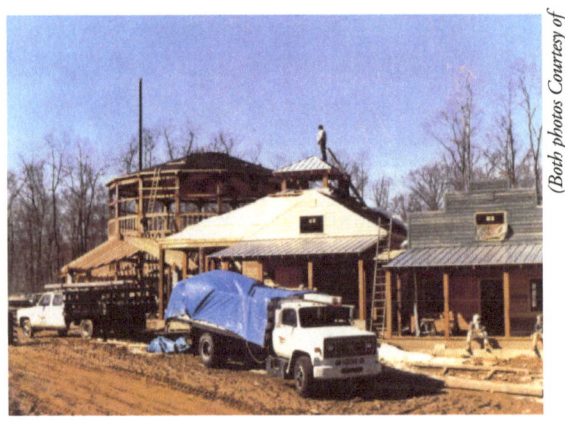

Construction of Arts & Crafts

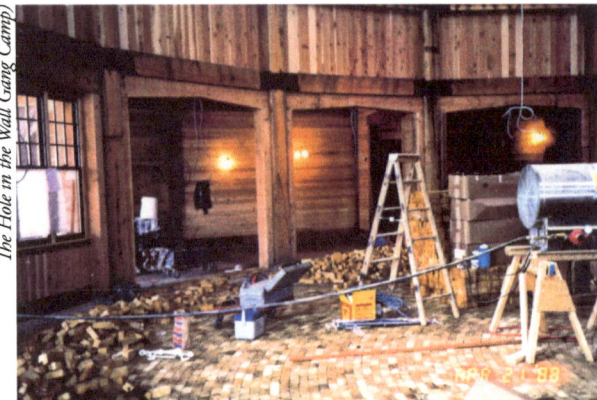

Construction of Dining Hall interior

(Both photos Courtesy of The Hole in the Wall Gang Camp)

Children with other bleeding disorders also benefit by these precautions. Over the years, several other summer camps have developed programs that allow this activity for boys with hemophilia.[4] The Professional Association of Therapeutic Horsemanship International (PATH), in its manual, "PATH International Standards for Certification and Accreditation," still lists horseback riding as a precaution for service and in severe cases, a contraindication due to bleeding risks of hemophilia.[5]

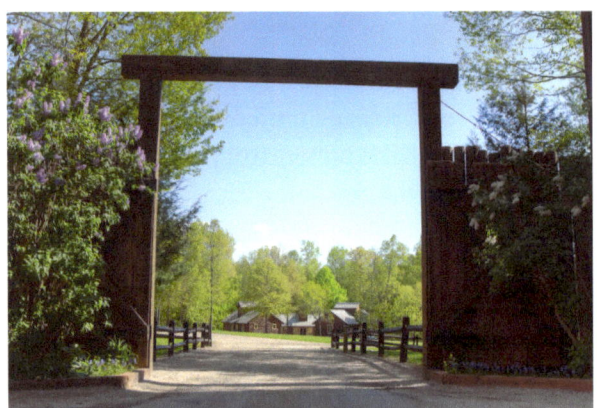

Entering the cabin circle

(Photo © Matthew Pearson)

The Infirmary was designed to maximize efficiency and accessibility. My long-time sickle cell nurse practitioner Sue Staples, whose name became Johnson when she married, and I met repeatedly with the architects in planning the Infirmary. Knowing that there would be campers receiving medications at mealtimes, the Infirmary was strategically located close to the Dining Hall, where all of the children would be together three times a day for meals. The layout and design of the Infirmary maximized convenience, safety and attractiveness. There was a central, secure pharmacy where medications were kept. There were originally two examination/treatment rooms and two rooms with beds where children could receive infusions or be observed for a period of time. There was an office for the nurses. For each camper, the nurses made a folder containing the application and a place for notes of any visits to the Infirmary for acute care. These folders were kept in an alphabetically arranged filing cabinet. At the end of the session, copies of the Infirmary notes were sent to the camper's doctor. For the first year, there were at least three or four nurses and two doctors each session. Living quarters for the nurses and doctors were attached to, but separate

---

4   Information on camps offering horseback riding to boys with hemophilia can be found on the National Hemophilia Foundation's website: www.hemophilia.org.

5   See www.pathintl.org/path-intl-membership/my-path-intl-membership/standards-manual (page 205 of the 2014 edition). The mission of PATH is to promote "safety and optimal outcomes in equine-assisted activities and therapies for individuals with special needs."

from, the Infirmary itself.

Dr. Anne (Annie) Dyson, a pediatrician and philanthropist, joined the Board at Paul's invitation in 1988. The Dyson Foundation, established by her parents, had paid for the construction of the Infirmary. Annie became Chair of the Board in 1997 and was a regular volunteer doctor over several summers until she passed away in 2000. At an early point, she held a contest to find a suitable name for the Infirmary; the winner was "The OK Corral."

On June 4, 1988, a dedication ceremony was held in the gymnasium during which Paul announced that he had renamed the man-made lake "Pearson Pond" in my honor. The last bulldozers and trucks left Camp the fourth week of May. Mike and Simon had miraculously seen to the completion of THITWGC's 35 new buildings and all of the infrastructure needs. The process—from the beginning of Camp design to construction completion—had taken only 18 months. Paul's deadline had been met! Two weeks later, the first campers arrived.

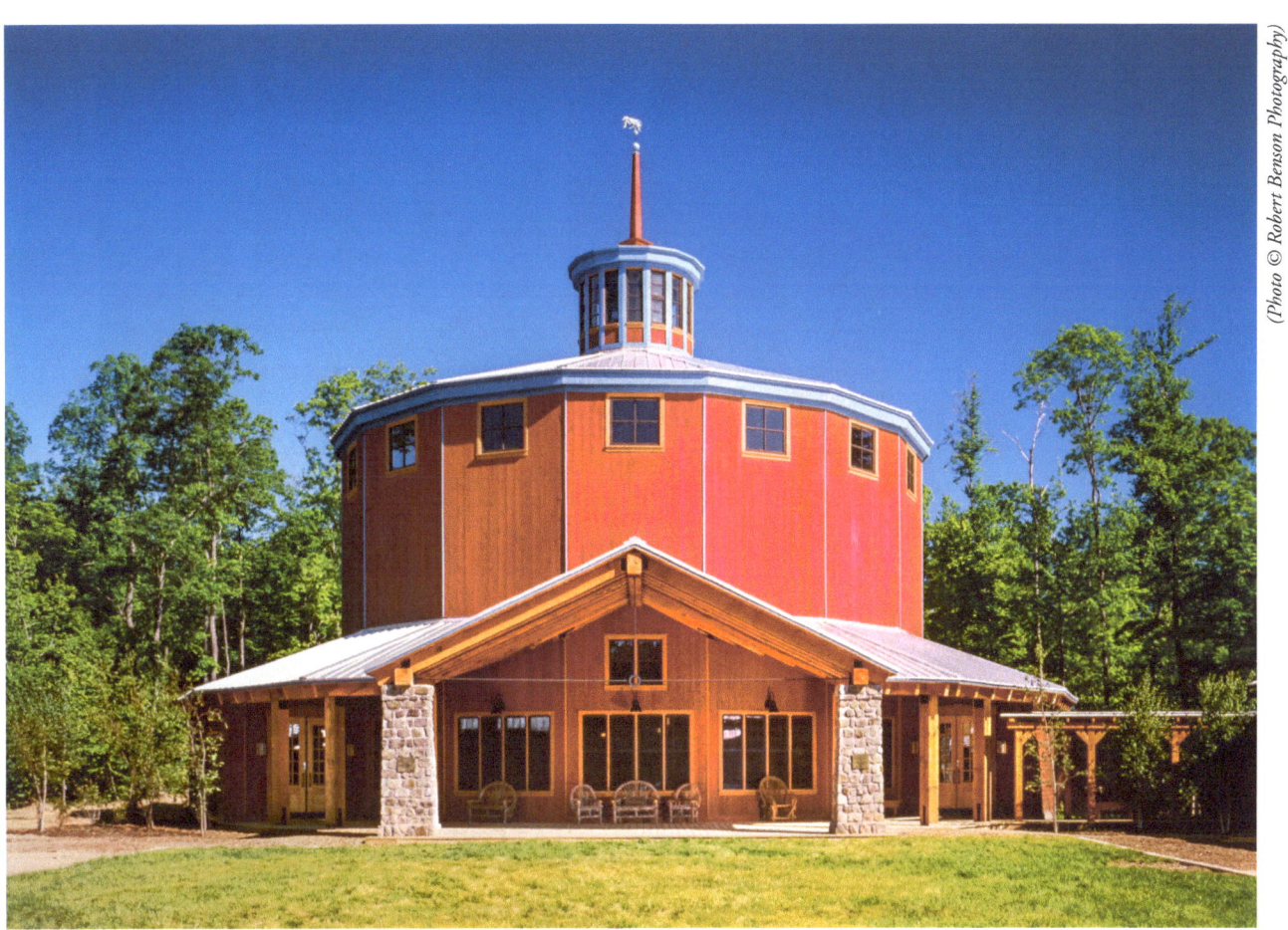

Dining Hall exterior

CHAPTER 2 ~ Camp Location, Design, and Construction

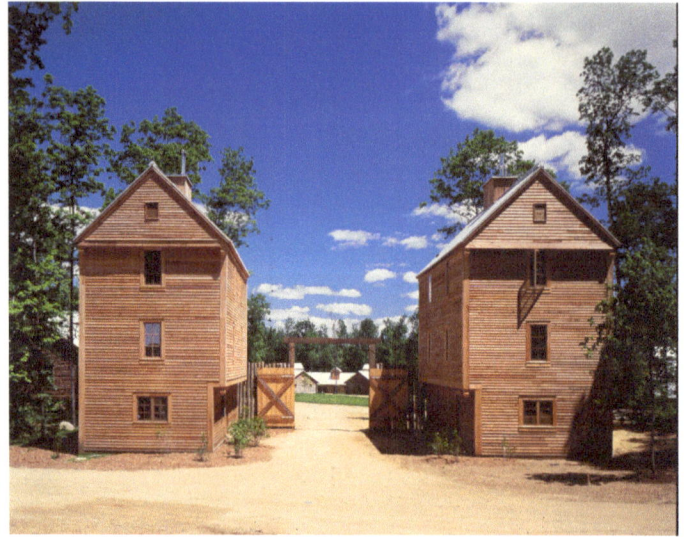

Cabin area entrance with stockades

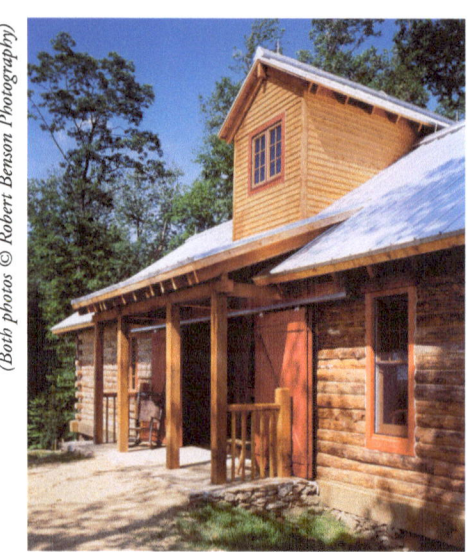

Completed cabin

(Both photos © Robert Benson Photography)

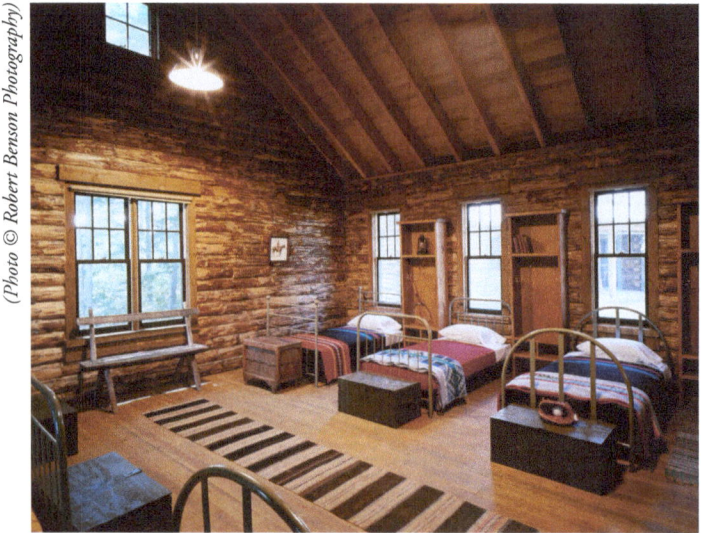

Cabin interior

(Photo © Robert Benson Photography)

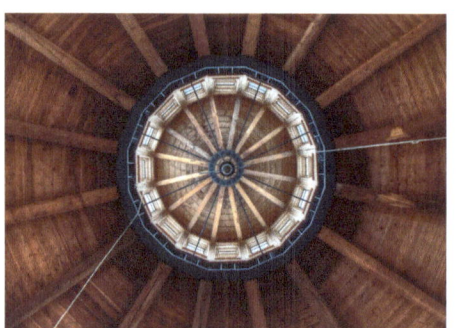

Dining Hall ceiling

(Photo © Matthew Pearson)

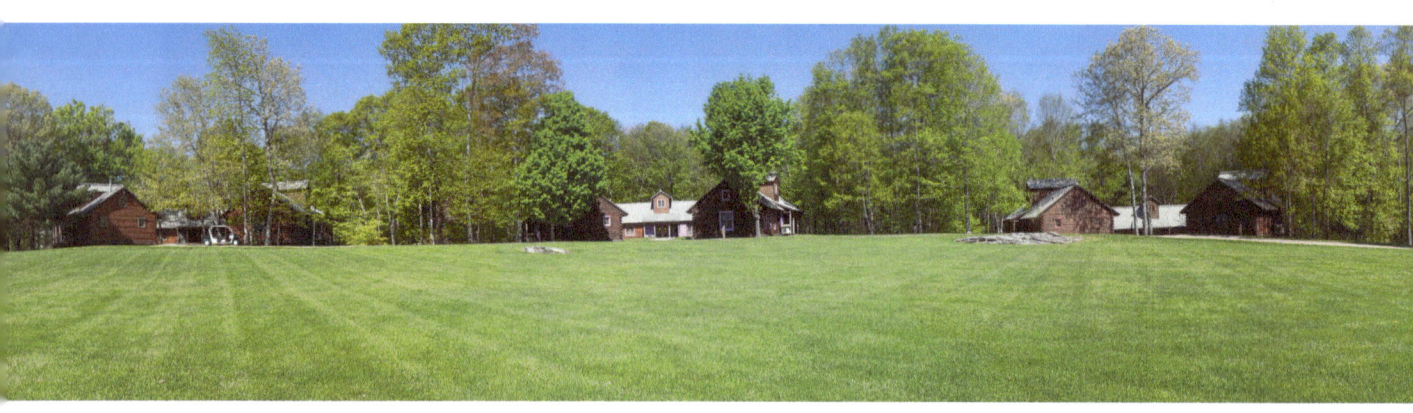

Cabin circle

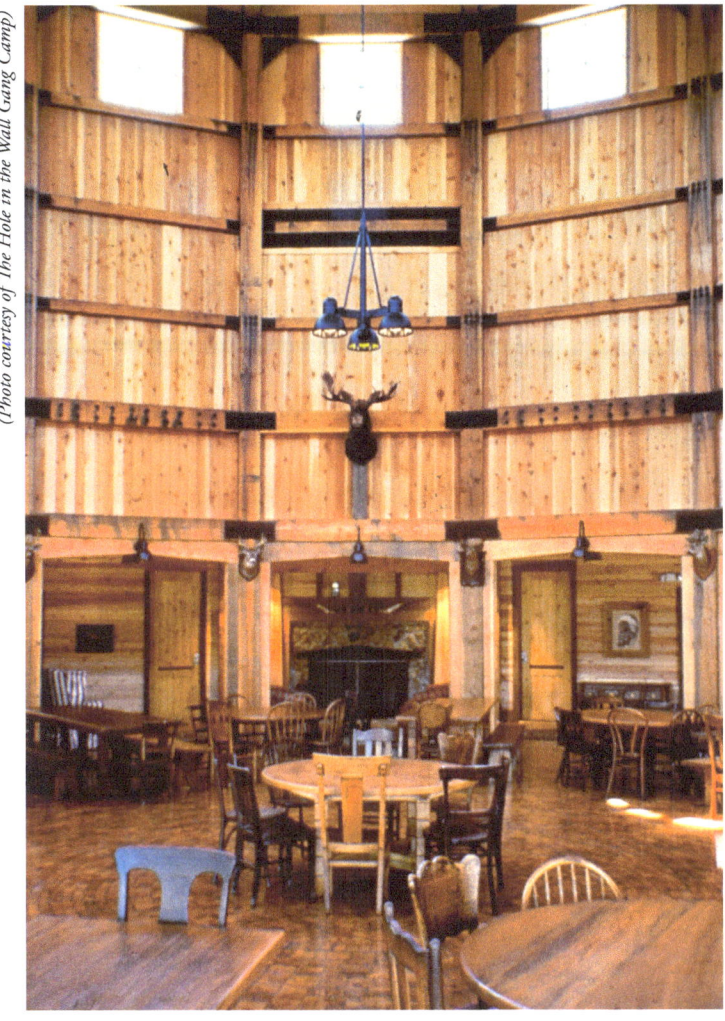

Dining Hall interior

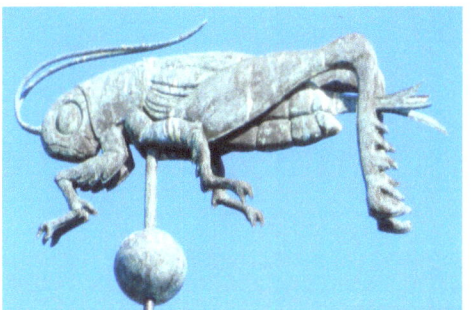

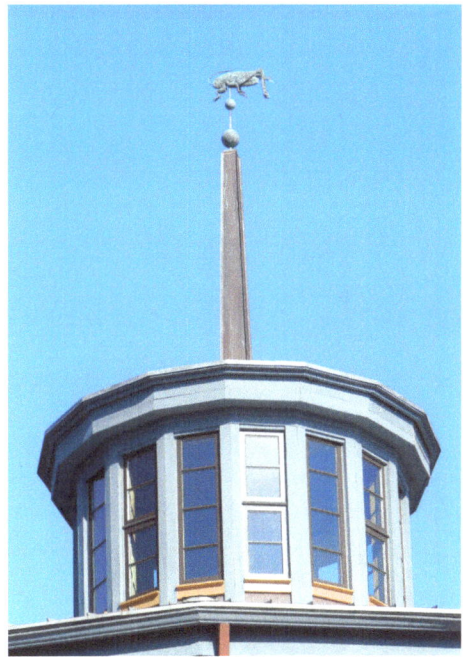

A cricket weather vane on top of Dining Hall

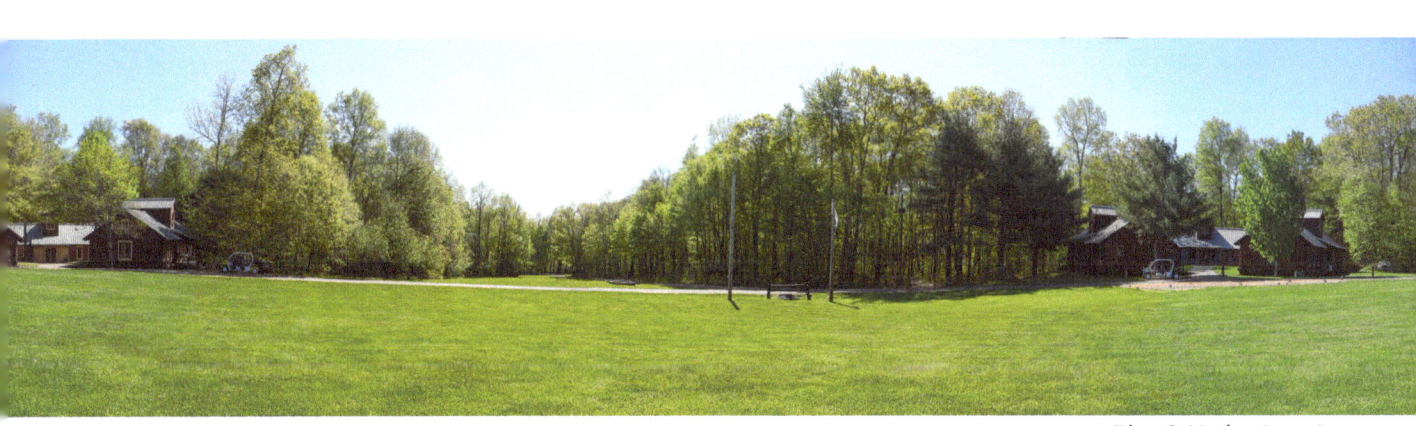

CHAPTER 2 ~ Camp Location, Design, and Construction

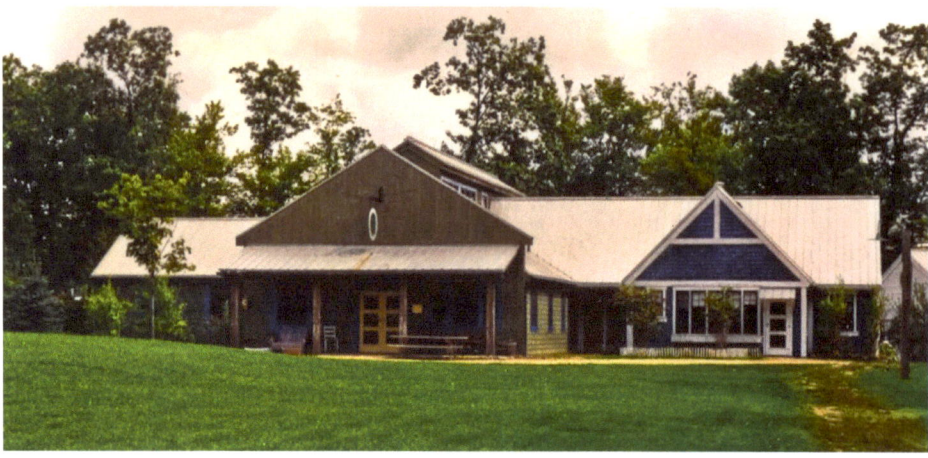

The OK Corral Infirmary and adjacent nursing quarters

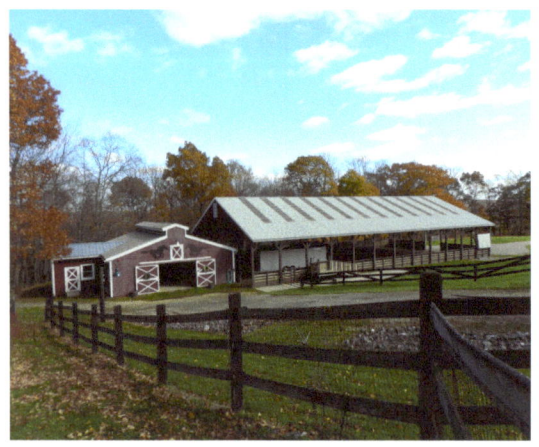

Horse Barn

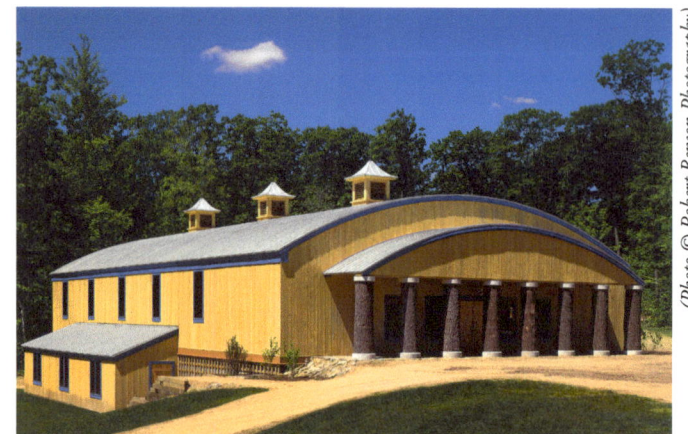

Gymnasium

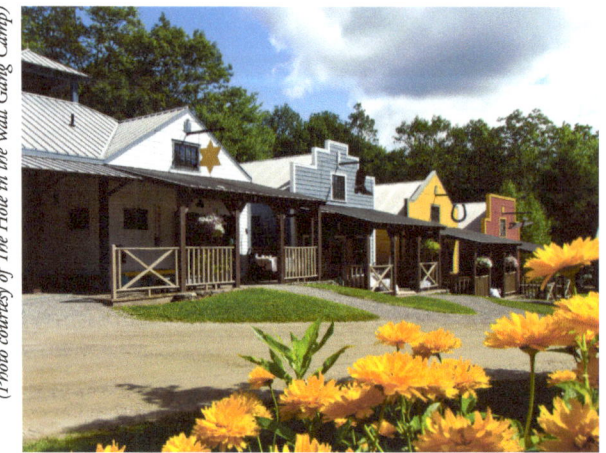

Arts & Crafts

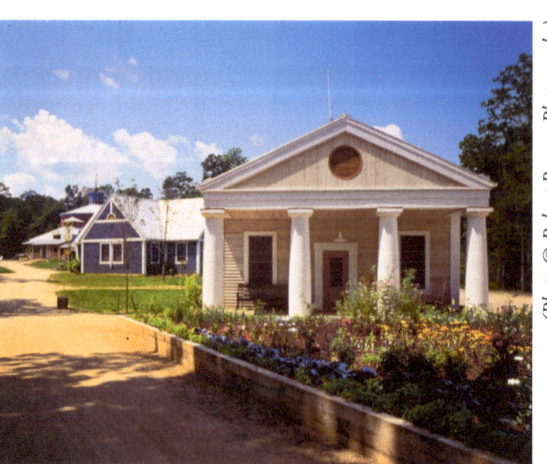

Administration building

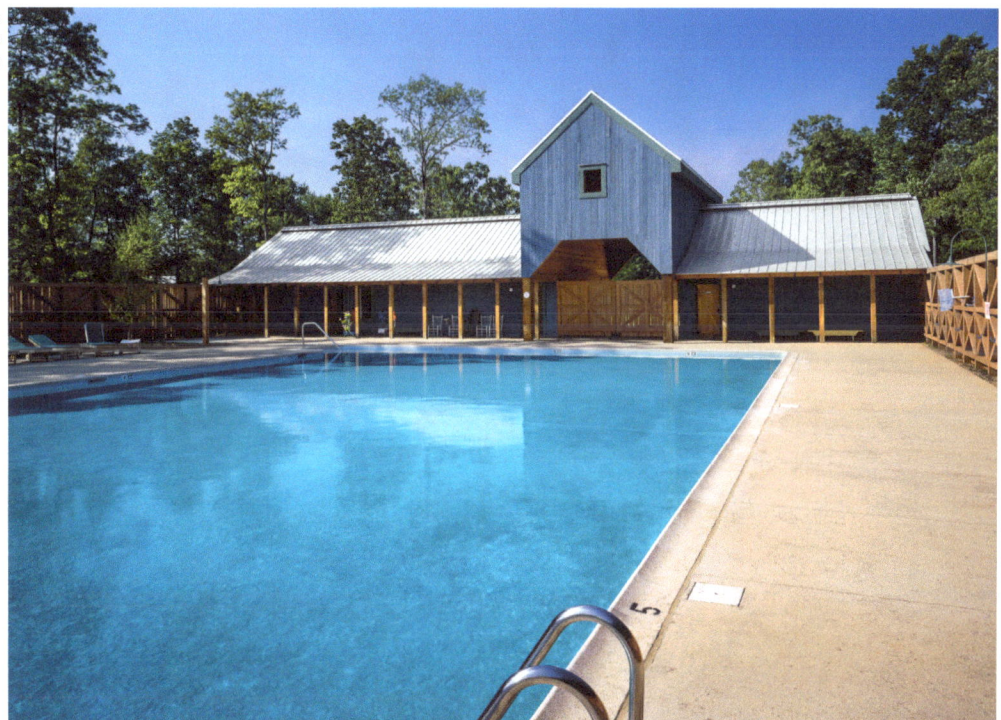

Swimming Pool

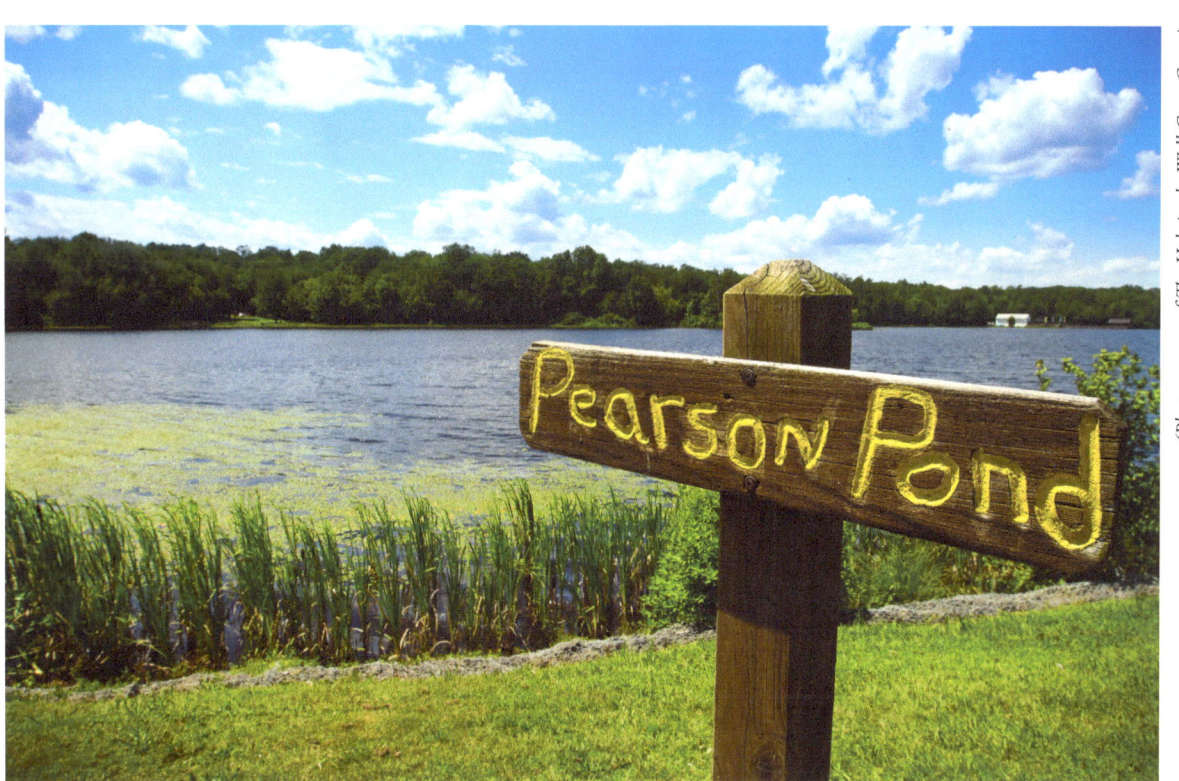

Pearson Pond

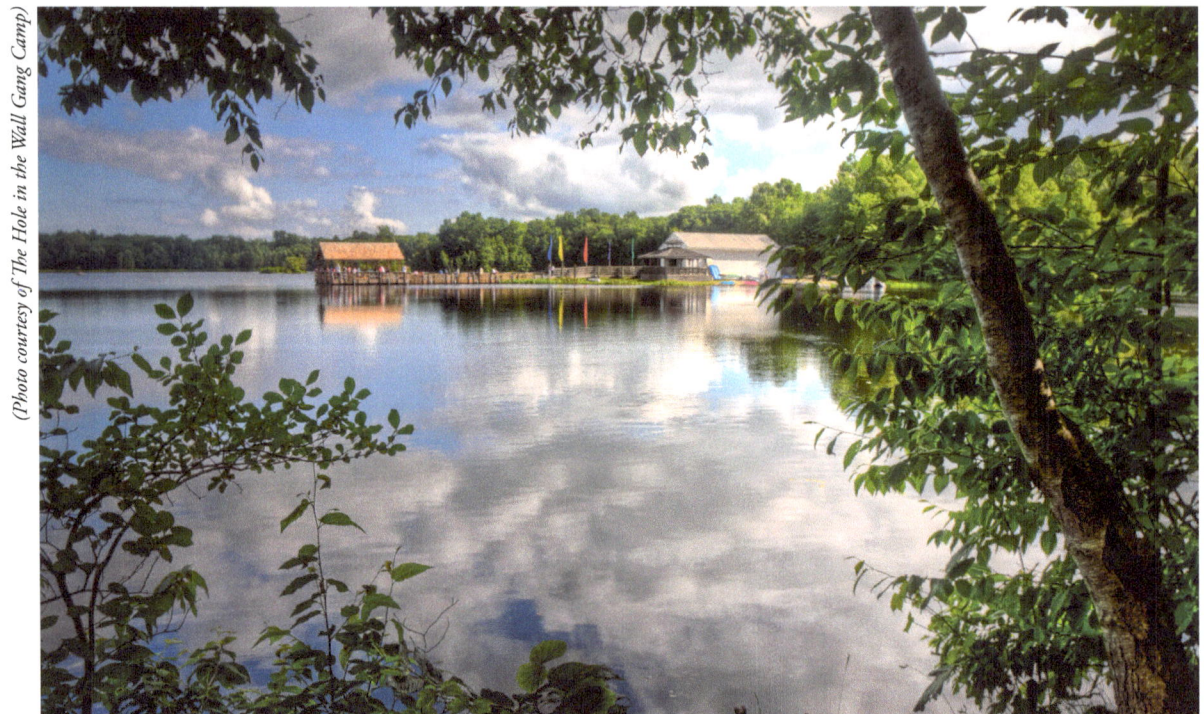

Boathouse on Pearson Pond

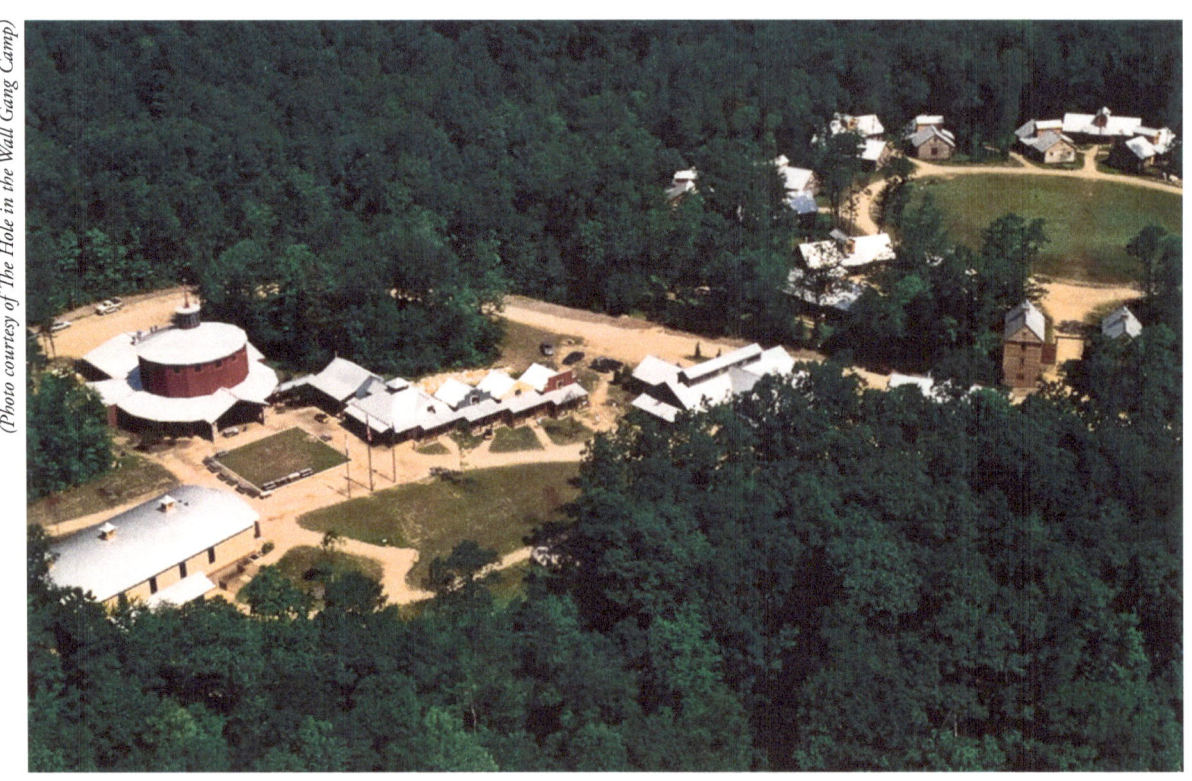

Aerial view of Camp, 1988

CHAPTER THREE

Recruiting Campers and Developing the Medical Program

While the physical structures were being developed, I began planning the medical aspects of THITWGC. To successfully recruit campers, I would have to convince the pediatric hematology/oncology community in New England as well as the parents of potential campers that Camp would be a safe place for medically fragile children. In the late 1960s in New Haven, I had the good fortune to meet Dorothy (Dotty) Guiliotis, a remarkable woman of Greek heritage who was involved in helping families with thalassemia, a genetic blood disease discussed later. Thalassemia had tragically affected Dotty's family. Her youngest sister, Georgene, had passed away from the disease in 1972 just before her 21st birthday. During the early days of planning, Dotty was uncertain that we could convince families to send their children with life-threatening diseases to a summer camp in the woods of northeastern Connecticut. She bluntly told me that her family would have been too protective to allow Georgene to attend a camp. Although Dotty was right much of the time, she admitted that she was wrong during her first visit to Camp. However, her initial concerns caused me to plan and promote Paul's dream cautiously and to enlist the strong support of the New England pediatric hematology/oncology community.

In the summer of 1987, I held a meeting to introduce the idea of THITWGC to New England's pediatric hematology/oncology clinic directors. We were a relatively small group—we all knew each other. By state, there were the following programs:

Connecticut:
- University of Connecticut School of Medicine, Hartford Hospital, Hartford
- Yale School of Medicine, Yale-New Haven Hospital, New Haven

Massachusetts:
- Harvard Medical School, Boston Children's Hospital, Boston

- Tufts Medical School, Floating Hospital, Boston
- Boston University Medical School, Boston Medical Center, Boston
- University of Massachusetts Medical School, University of Massachusetts Medical Center, Worcester

Rhode Island:
- Alpert School of Medicine at Brown University, Hasboro Children's Hospital, Providence

New Hampshire:
- Dartmouth Medical School at Mary Hitchcock Hospital, Hanover

I invited each of these clinics to send a representative to the meeting, which was held in Paul's barn. Invitations went out on Paul Newman's stationery, which I am sure captured the attention of the invitees! We had 100% turnout of directors or their representatives at the meeting. I summarized the plans for Camp and showed them the architect's scale model.

Their response was enthusiastic and supportive. Although the detailed medical coverage had not been determined, I promised them that there would be competent on-site supervision and care for the children. There would be well-defined procedures in place to meet emergencies that might arise. Because I had their trust, my colleagues said that they would try to recruit their patients as campers and tell their families that THITWGC would be a safe place for their children. In this way, I attempted to overcome the concerns expressed by Dotty and others that parents might be reluctant to relinquish their medically-fragile children to Camp. Later, when we were up and running, some of these colleagues participated as volunteer physicians.

A few months after this Westport meeting, in an effort to begin recruitment, I brought Sue Staples actively into the medical program development. Together, Sue and I began to do what was needed to make things work. We started by developing the application and distributing copies for potential campers through the pediatric hematology/oncology programs in New England. These applications required a medical summary, a list of medications with any special instructions, and a signed permission from a parent allowing THITWGC to dispense medication to campers and provide medical care while on site.

In the spring of 1988, I became increasingly concerned about the medical and nursing coverage at Camp. The recently hired Camp Director repeatedly told me, "Don't worry, I've got it under control." In June, just two weeks before the first campers were scheduled to arrive, he again told me everything was under control. My commitment to colleagues to make Camp a safe place for medically fragile children had prompted me to personally prepare alternatives for their medical needs throughout the planning process. Because of the Director's reluctance to share any obvious plan with me, I was well prepared to do whatever was needed. Forty-eight hours before it was to open, Sue and I went to Camp and bluntly asked the Director, "What is the medical and nursing coverage going to be?" His response was, "I have my wife who is an LPN (licensed practical nurse)." He apparently did not realize that LPNs cannot work without direct medical supervision and cannot dispense many medications. Because of promises to physicians and families that there would be adequate on-site medical and nursing coverage, I said to Sue, "It looks like we are here for the summer." With no hesitation, we moved ourselves into the doctors' and nurses' quarters.

I was at THITWGC full time for the next 14 summers, while Sue was there for 12. Although this was more personal participation than I had anticipated, I was able to do it because I was a senior, tenured professor at Yale and did not have to worry about promotion. I scheduled necessary departmental and clinical work in New Haven during the two-day inter-sessions. I am grateful to my departmental colleagues—among them were Doctors Norm Siegel, Dick O'Brien, Kim Ritchie, Mike Genel, and Joe Zelson—who covered for me while I was at Camp. My secretary, Ann Marie Anderson, communicated with me daily about what I needed to do for Yale while at Camp, and she helped me maintain a long-distance presence in the Pediatric Department. Sue was able to be at Camp because she was my sickle cell nurse practitioner. Since we were still employees of Yale Medical School, our medical liability was covered. There was an adjustment for my family as well. My wife Anne spent a good deal of time at Camp, although she occasionally reminded me that we had not attended the Boston Symphony summer concerts at Tanglewood for many years.

The contributions of Sue from the initial planning stages and throughout the first 12 years of THITWGC cannot be overestimated. She was instrumental in camper selection. During the spring of 1988, applications began to trickle in. We reviewed them and called families to answer any questions and to reassure them about the medical support services we would provide. Although priority was given to children with cancer and serious blood diseases, we accepted children with other diagnoses if it were likely that they could not attend an ordinary camp. Sue developed systems for checking children in and out of Camp. She established the procedures for dispensing medications and conducting sick calls. She recruited staff and volunteer nurses who were assigned to the individual Units. During these years, Sue married and had two children who spent the summers with her at THITWGC.

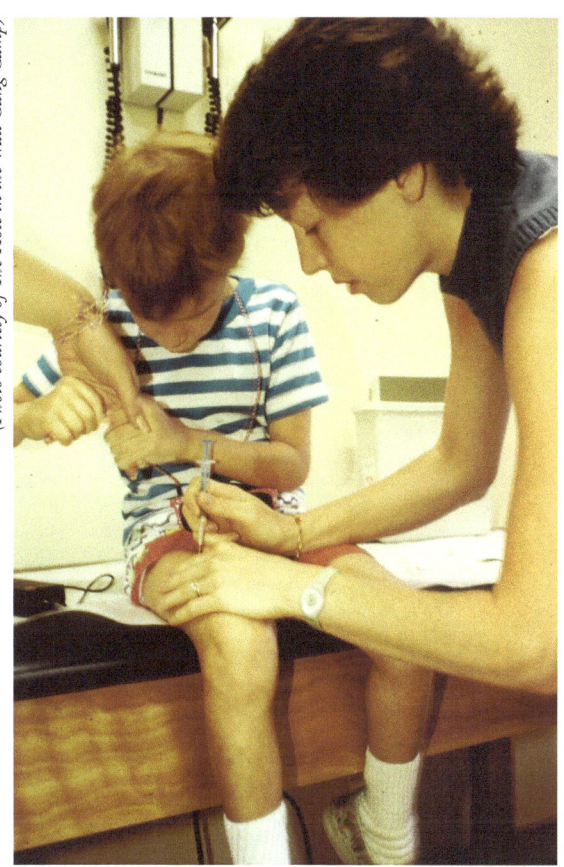

(Photo courtesy of The Hole in the Wall Gang Camp)

Nursing Director Sue Johnson treating a camper in the Infirmary

Sue and I put together the medical and nursing programs so that we were able to do things that cannot be done at an ordinary camp. In addition to on-site processes and procedures for handling medically complicated children, we made arrangements with nearby Windham and Day Kimball Hospitals for laboratory and X-ray services. We compiled a long list of medications that I gave to the Yale-New Haven Hospital pharmacy, which stocked our Infirmary inventory.

We established criteria for the transport of children who might need to leave Camp because of medical complications. We developed protocols to have these children transferred back to their home hospitals as a first preference. Each summer, a small number had to be evacuated, most often because of a severe sickle cell pain crisis or fever in a child with neutropenia (a low white blood cell count, which puts the child at a risk for having a serious infection). Although it was fortunately never necessary, I made back-up arrangements for emergency helicopter evacuations to Yale-New Haven Hospital of a critically ill child. No child has ever died at THITWGC, although there have been some near misses. These were due to complications of their diseases and not due to accidents or something we could have prevented. Our detailed advance planning and adjustments during these years reaped rewards in achieving a safe and supportive medical environment that allowed campers to maximize their time having fun together.

While Sue and I were busy preparing the necessary medical and nursing support for campers, others were busy planning and developing all of the fun Camp activities. Counselors and support staff were hired and trained, volunteers were recruited, furnishings and supplies were purchased, and THITWGC was made ready for campers. It was a stunning, breath-taking place that would deal with tears, homesickness, and pain through the array of activities, laughter, enthusiasm, empathy, support, growth, joy, and celebration.

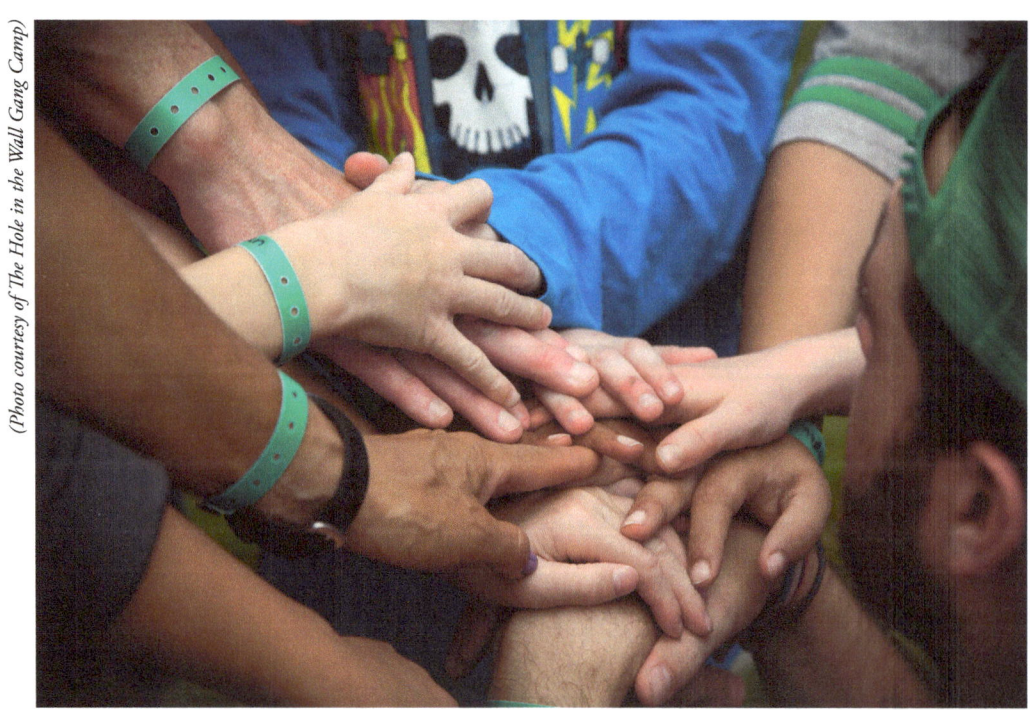

(Photo courtesy of The Hole in the Wall Gang Camp)

CHAPTER FOUR

Additions After Camp's Opening

As programs continued to evolve after Camp's opening in 1988, new needs were identified. We developed ways to meet and address those needs. The first additional area became known as the Memory Garden. After the first session, a spontaneous gathering of staff took place in a quiet outdoor area near where the Tower (see below) is now located after news came that a camper, Philip, had died shortly after returning home. Philip had been very ill while at Camp but had enjoyed the experience to the maximum. His parents were grateful that Philip had the opportunity to attend. I assured the staff that his experience at Camp had not hastened his death; rather, it had provided joy to both Philip and his family. Someone built a campfire as staff gathered together. Bob (Woody) Wilkins, who worked at THITWGC from 1988 to 1993, first as Wood Shop Director and then as Camp Director for two years, placed a big log near the campfire so that staff had a place to set candles and light them. For some on the staff, it was their first reality that campers could die from their diseases. They quickly realized that they needed a special place for working through their grief together by talking, sharing memories, meditating, and praying. The Memory Garden became that place and is still in use today to remember those who have passed away and to provide comfort.

After Camp opened and camper numbers were increasing, we realized that extra hand washing capacity was needed at the Dining Hall. As a result, a long trough for hand washing was installed at the entrance door.

As the planning for Camp buildings had progressed in 1986-87, the projected costs escalated. This worried some Board members, and they made decisions to scale down somewhat. In spite of Hotch's vigorous protest, plans for a theater were shelved because a majority of the Board believed that the Dining Hall could be used for skits and evening programs. During the summer of 1988, it became apparent that the Dining Hall could not effectively serve as a theater substitute. Program rehearsals could not easily take place during the day because of meal preparation and clean up. Furthermore, the Dining Hall had not been designed with the appropriate space and acoustics for skits and performances. Hotch, feeling very strongly that a theater was necessary, had Mike Kolakowski dig a big, deep hole near the Dining Hall. At the next Board meeting when Hotch again brought up the need for a theater, the other Board members conceded, "Well, maybe it's something to think about." Hotch responded, "It better be soon because there's a big hole that's going to fill up with water and become an attractive nuisance that a child could fall into." This potential hazard caused the Board to make a theater a high priority.

In 1989, Tom and his architects designed the Theater, modeled after a western honky-tonk music hall. It was built and opened in 1990 to accommodate about 280 people. Theater accessibility is so natural and seamless that a child in a wheelchair can easily enter the front door, have a place to watch a presentation, and maneuver to onstage and backstage in a few moments without stairs to negotiate. It soon became a focal point of Camp and has been well used over the years. Five years after it was built, the Theater was enlarged to add more space for rehearsals and meetings.

Expansion of the medical and nursing staff in following years was necessitated by an increase in the number of campers. In 1995, Doc's House was built a short distance from the Infirmary to provide accommodations for the physicians and volunteer medical staff, including medical students, pediatric residents, and fellows in pediatric hematology/oncology. Each of the two wings has a master bedroom with private bath and two other bedrooms with a shared bathroom. I moved from the back of the Infirmary to one of the wings. The Infirmary itself underwent major revisions in 1994 and 1995, and a nursing staff house (referred to as the "Chalet") was constructed three years later. The size of the pharmacy was increased to accommodate the volume of medications dispensed. The examining rooms were increased to five. These rooms were

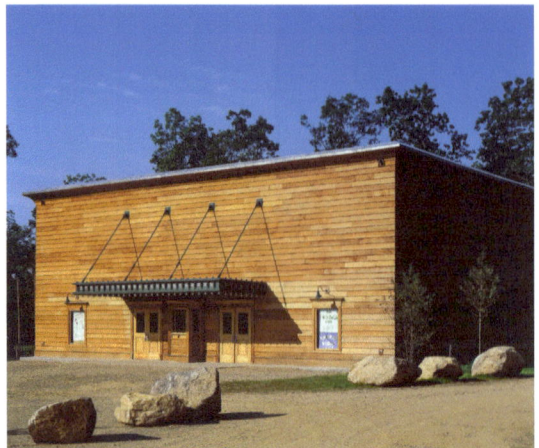

Theater exterior

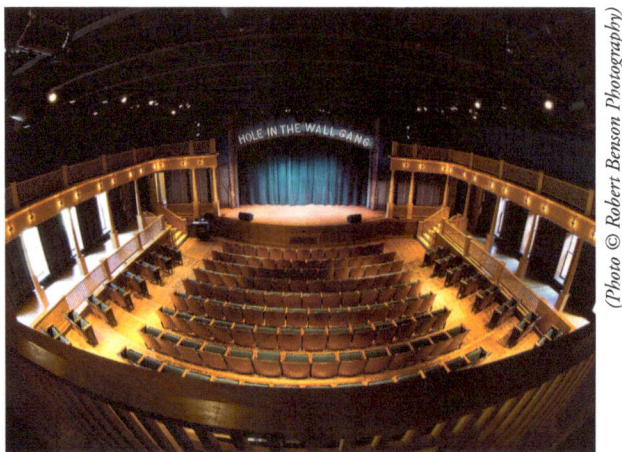

Theater interior

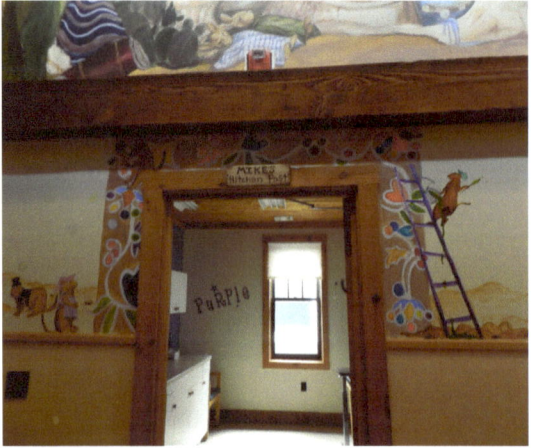

Purple Unit exam room

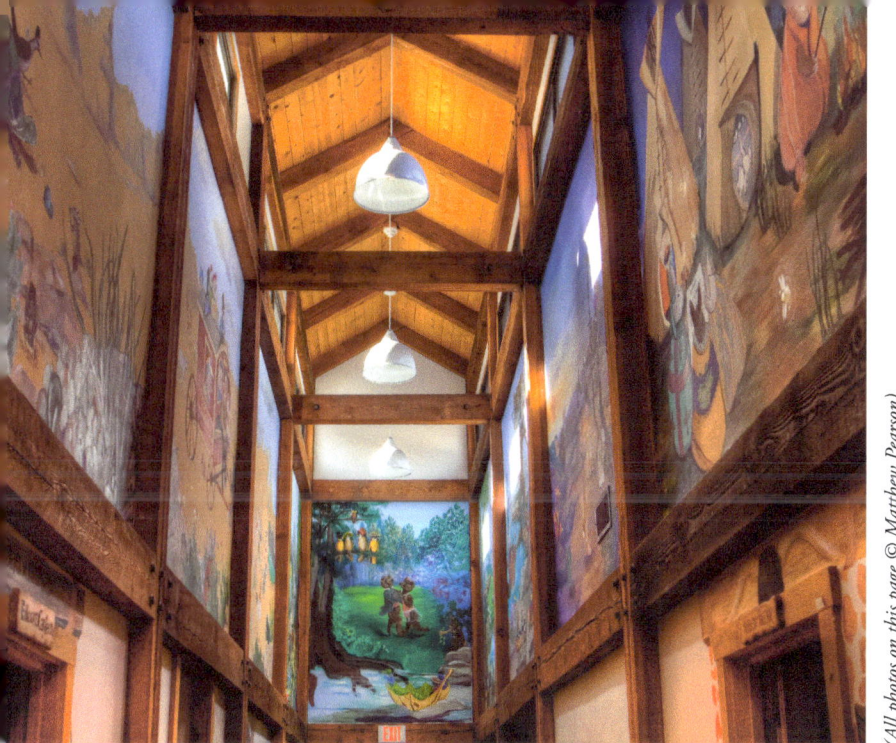

Main Infirmary vaulted hallway lined with Sherry's murals

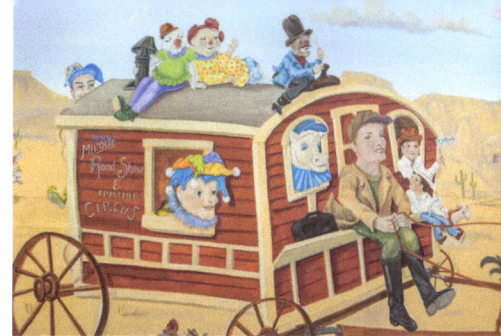

Clown-filled circus wagon driven by Annie Dyson

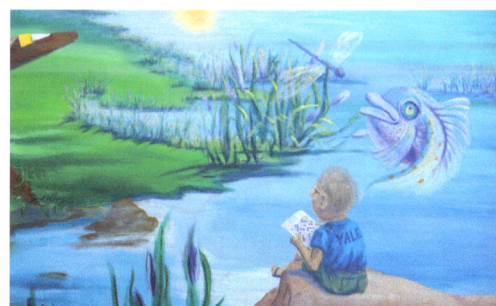

My caricature working on a crossword puzzle by Pearson Pond, with jumping Wee-Pee

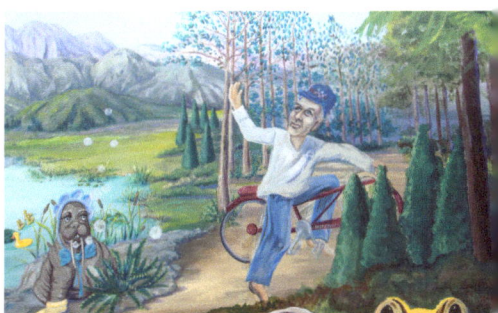

Paul riding his bicycle

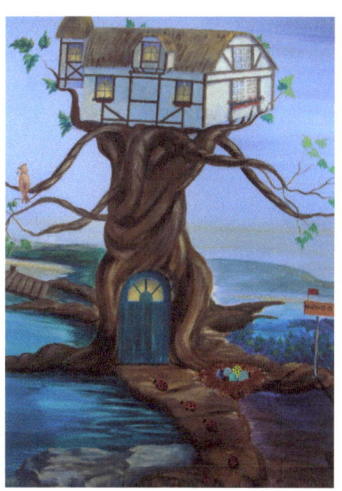

Sherry's mural of the Tree House

assigned to the individual Units and were staffed by the Unit nurses. Enclosing the existing front porch increased the waiting area space. Colorful decorations and furniture along with toys and books in the waiting area were added to make the Infirmary a welcoming, non-hospital-looking place.

Over the years, Camp Artist Sherry Talley painted a number of colorful murals in segmented panels on the high walls of the Infirmary, making it a warm, comforting, and entertaining environment. In one panel, Dr. Annie Dyson is driving a circus wagon full of clowns. In another, I am shown wearing a Yale t-shirt while working on a crossword puzzle, one of my favorite pastimes. As I sit on a rock overlooking Pearson Pond, I can see the mystical, ephemeral fish Wee-Pee jumping from beneath the surface. Another mural depicts Paul riding his bicycle, which he often did at Camp. It is reminiscent of the scene in *Butch Cassidy and the Sundance Kid* with Butch (played by Paul) on a bicycle riding to the tune of the Oscar-winning song "Raindrops Keep Fallin' on My Head." The panel that depicts a house on top of a tree represents the Tree House (explained later) and has a mailbox with "NewMoose" (a take-off on Paul's last name) on it. Lucky ladybugs are marching past a bird's nest with eggs and toward the tree.

As other needs were identified during the first few years, Camp responded in creative and all-inclusive ways. The Ropes Challenge Course was professionally designed and installed beginning in 1992 to provide three levels of challenge activities that promote group cooperation, communication, collaboration, and the building of individual self-esteem. It had been noticed in the early years that there were a small number of children in each session with significant physical limitations struggling to participate in some of the activities. Woody, who was Camp Director at the time, led the efforts to have a Low Ropes Challenge Course installed first, which would allow the participation of all campers. Medium and High Challenges were added afterwards. These three levels allowed collaborative group activities ranging from simple to complicated. The professional group Northeast Adventures built the Challenge Course and provided staff training.

Dr. Sam Ross wanted more than just horses at Camp. It has been known for over 25 years that interaction with animals, such as petting a dog, has healing effects on humans and can reduce blood pressure[1] and anxiety. In addition, it can enhance feelings of self-worth and decrease social isolation.[2] Two lovable, calm Labrador Retrievers—Yellow Lab Kaly and Black Lab Dukey—lived at Camp while Woody was Camp Director.[3] Both dogs could be seen roaming the area with staff, constantly asking for attention with their soft, expressive eyes and wagging tails. With Sam's urging and support, George Harakaly brought in some domesticated animals such as goats, sheep, chickens, ponies, and Vietnamese pot-bellied pigs, some of which came from the farm at Green Chimneys. As a result, campers who tired easily had an observational activity that provided comfort, relaxation, and animal companionship in a peaceful atmosphere. The original animal area was located behind the Theater near the center part of Camp. It was later moved near the Horse Barn in order to allow the animals to be cared for by the equestrian staff, but it was eventually phased out as more convenient activity options proliferated closer to the center of Camp than the Horse Barn.

Newman's Nook was constructed as an amphitheater for group programs. It featured a stone wall with a hole, at the base of which is a white stone that Paul brought back from Butch Cassidy's hideout at the Hole in the Wall Pass in Wyoming.

Facing physical challenges and successfully meeting them can provide people with

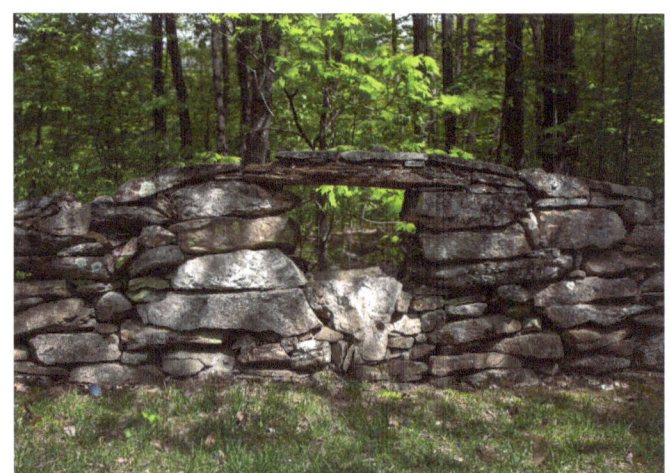

Newman's Nook at the campfire circle, featuring the white stone from Wyoming

(Photo © Matthew Pearson)

---

1 Vormbrock JK, Grossberg JM, "Cardiovascular effects of human-pet dog interactions." *J Behav Med.* 1988 Oct;11(5):509-17.
2 Wells, DL. "The effects of animals on human health and well-being." *Journal of Social Issues*, 2009; 65(3): 523-543.
3 Woody continues his work with hospitalized children through the nonprofit organization that he founded called Dances With Wood. His programs use woodworking to empower and inspire children who are battling cancer and other serious illnesses. The DWW program has been used in 33 hospitals in 26 states. He has also developed a healthcare education program for children with bleeding disorders that has been used in 23 summer camps around the USA. For more information, see www.danceswithwood.org.

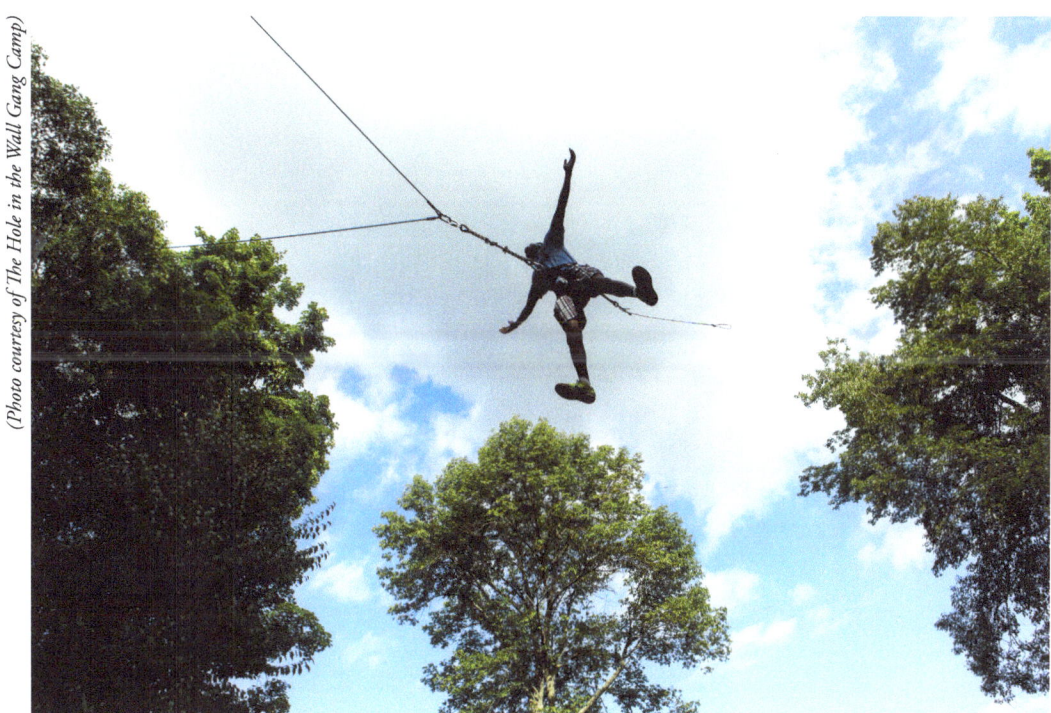
(Photo courtesy of The Hole in the Wall Gang Camp)

Soaring down on the zip line

an adrenaline surge followed by smug satisfaction. The Ropes Challenge Course had been successful, and we did not stop there. In 1996, Northeast Adventures built the Tower for rock-climbing simulation and installed the zip line, a speedy way to descend from the Tower, for memorable challenges and thrills so that older campers might have something special. Staff and volunteers are also offered an opportunity to scale to the top. Northeast Adventures complies with standards set by the Association of Challenge Course Technology and provides trainings and workshops to optimize safety. As is the process with each climber, when I met the Tower challenge, I was prepared for the experience by donning a helmet, getting connected with safety ropes, and going through the routine safety checklist step by step, including the exchange between Tower staff and climber: "Do you trust us?" "Yes, I trust you!" The cheers of people on the ground give many climbers the extra boost they need to reach the Tower top. Gentle tugging with the safety ropes can also help.

    The Tower is a focal point of cheering support and personal accomplishment. Some staff members have made their climbs extra challenging—I have seen a few of them

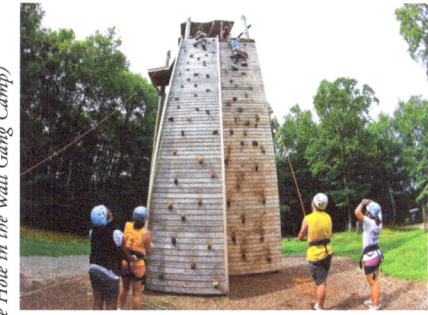

The Tower

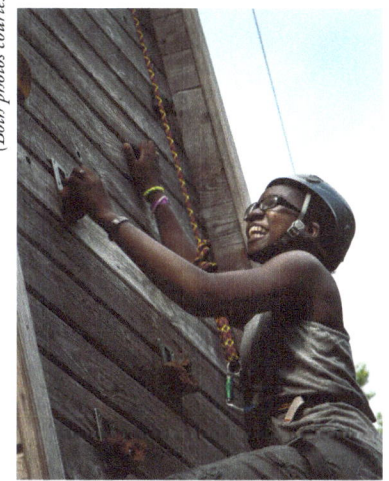

(Both photos courtesy of The Hole in the Wall Gang Camp)

Climbing the Tower

climb blindfolded as they were guided by someone on the ground with careful verbal directions for moving each arm and leg to attain the top. And Dan (Cappy) Capobianco from the Wood Shop climbed with only his arms. All of us who have done it can agree that it is both thrilling and satisfying! The Tower provides campers, who have undergone unpleasant physical challenges due to their illnesses, with an exhilarating physical accomplishment. The swooping descent on the zip line can provide a camper with a soaring sense of freedom.

The large Tree House, built with a donation from the Discover Card office in Westport and opened in 2003, has a meandering wheelchair accessible ramp. Special activities and meetings are frequently held there among the treetops.

Somewhat later, Lulu's Lodge and Steve's Station were constructed across the road and down the hill from the Swimming Pool. These both provide lodging rooms and meeting space. Program staff members room there during the summer. These winterized facilities provide adequate space for Parent Weekends and Camper Reunions in the spring and fall. The Lodge is named after long-time Camp supporter Andy Crowley's mother Lulu, and the Crowley family donated the construction money. Steve Ruchafsky covered the cost of Steve's Station.

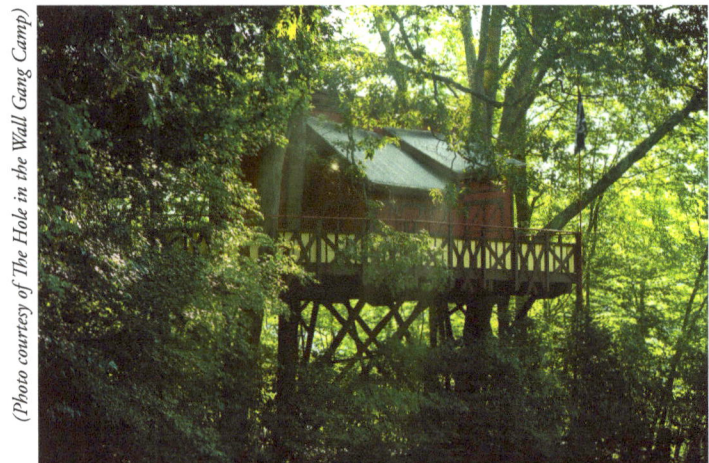

The Tree House

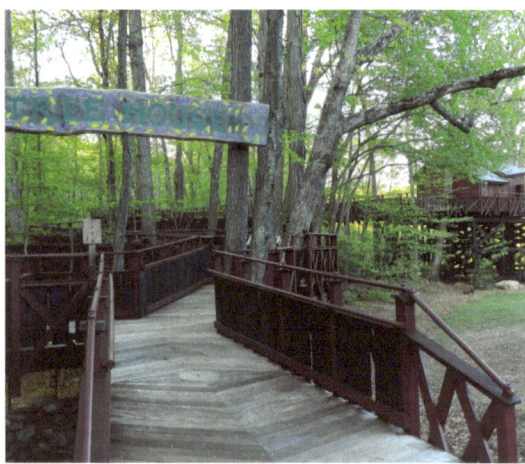

Ramp to the Tree House

CHAPTER FIVE

Laughter, Music, Dancing, Creativity, and Emotional Healing

From the start, the presence of the physicians and nurses made it possible for campers to continue the therapies prescribed by their pediatricians and hematologists/oncologists while they experienced the fun and laughter of THITWGC. However, Camp became much more than the traditional activities of a summer camping experience involving swimming, boating, fishing, and arts and crafts. Most people, when they visit THITWGC for the first time, detect a special feeling in the air—something that might be described as a combination of high positive energy, vibrations, and an electric feeling that might be termed as crazy or magical. It feels good to be there! Laughter, singing, dancing, and positive attitudes are contagious and work together to help children heal emotionally. Staff members make the magic happen—they are creative, energetic people with positive attitudes and an enormous capacity for giving and loving.

Research studies have shown that laughter can help relieve pain by increasing endorphins, which are natural painkillers. Laughter also reduces stress and enhances the quality of life, among other things.[1] Journalist and author Norman Cousins wrote about how laughter and a positive attitude helped him when he was seriously ill in the mid-1960s: "I made the joyous discovery that ten minutes of genuine belly laughter had an anesthetic effect and would give me at least two hours of pain-free sleep," he reported. "When the pain-killing effect of the laughter wore off, we would switch on the motion picture projector again and not infrequently, it would lead to another pain-free interval."[2] Laughing while watching Marx Brothers films and television comedies helped

---

1   http://www.cancercenter.com/treatments/laughter-therapy/ -- Cancer Treatment Centers of Amcrica wcbsitc
2   http://en.wikipedia.org/wiki/Norman_Cousins

Norman Cousins with his pain.[3]

Laughter is an omnipresent and vital component that has developed and evolved at Camp over the years, in large part due to the Big Apple Circus clowns. When children arrive for a session, they enter the property from Highway 44 onto a dirt road, pass underneath the rustic twig sign, and are greeted by enthusiastic staff and clowns dressed in costumes and brandishing water pistols. Starting from the first moments, the clowns infuse Camp with a mixture of imagination, exaggeration, expression, tricks, whimsy, silliness, and laughter. Along with the other staff, the clowns create a general atmosphere that lifts campers' spirits and helps them emotionally soar. The clowns are professionals from the nonprofit Big Apple Circus (BAC) in New York City, founded in 1977 by Paul Binder and Michael Christensen as a classical European-style, one-ring circus dedicated to serving the communities in which they perform. Opening their first show in a small green canvas tent pitched on the Battery City landfill in the shadow of the World Trade Center, the BAC presented world-class equestrian, juggling, acrobatic, and clown acts. Partnering with Moscow State Circus veteran performers and teachers Gregory Fedin and Nina Krasavina, they also created the New York School for Circus Arts as part of their commitment to serving the community.

Inspired by the death of his brother from pancreatic cancer, Michael Christensen created the BAC Clown Care® in 1986. This innovative community outreach program places professional performers into pediatric hospitals. These "clown doctors" integrate juggling, mime, music, storytelling, puppetry, magic, and slapstick into their "clown rounds," to reducing stress for children, caregivers, and medical staff they serve. Each artist goes through a rigorous training process to adapt their artistic specialty for the hospital enviornment and to comply with infection control protocols. Aligning themselves with the positive aspects of the children, nurturing feelings of wonder, awe, triumph and celebration, this remarkable program has inspired a worldwide profession known as hospital clowning. The BAC still gives circus performances and provides other community service programs in the Northeast.[4]

In 2014, Clown Care had 80 Clown Doctors working with hospitalized children in 16 pediatric facilities, where they conducted their special "clown rounds" and prescribed the power of humor for healing. Dr. John M. Driscoll Jr., former Chairman of the Pediatric Department at Morgan Stanley Children's Hospital of Columbia Presbyterian Medical Center in New York City, has aptly described the work of Clown Care: "Ministering to sick children goes beyond medication and technology. When a child begins to laugh it means he's probably beginning to feel better. I see the clowns as healers."[5]

Paul Newman had been an active supporter of the BAC and its Clown Care program through Newman's Own Foundation. While the circus was performing in Boston in June 1988, Michael, along with that year's production star Yang Xio Di and veteran Clown Care artist Kim Winslow, joined Paul and the staff on the opening day of The Hole in the Wall Gang Camp. Through these three artists, the BAC and its Clown Care program became a perfect partner of

3   http://www.laughingdiva.com/2012/12/how-laughter-therapy-cured-norman-cousins-of-a-life-threatening-form-of-arthritis/
4   https://en.wikipedia.org/wiki/Big_Apple_Circus; personal communication with Michael Christensen; and http://bigapplecircus.org/
5   http://bigapplecircus.org/clown-care

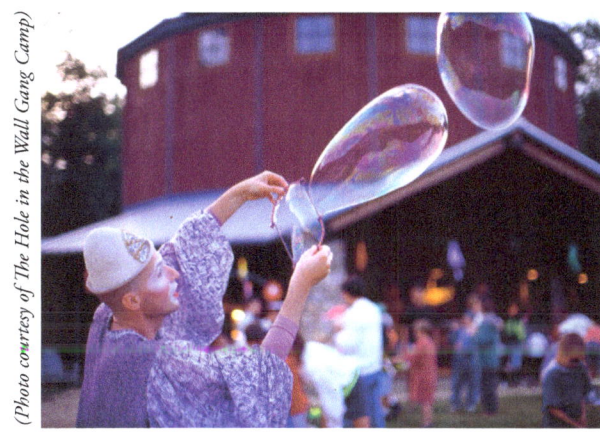

Kim/Loon blowing bubbles in front of the Dining Hall

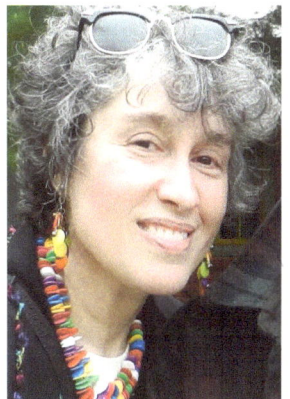

Ilene/Noodle, 2013

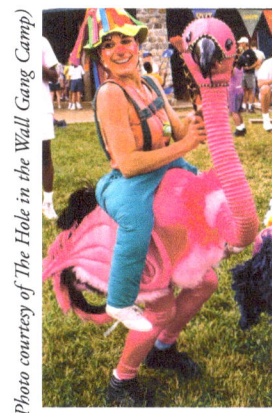

Fidget and Flora

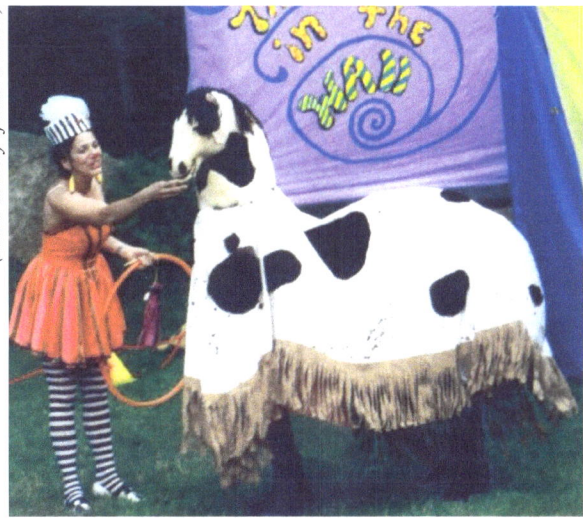

I am the rear end of Wonky the Wonder Horse with clown Hilary Chaplain as the trainer

THITWGC. Since 1989, the BAC has had resident pairs of clowns at Camp. Kim Winslow, whose clown name is "Loon," became known for skillfully blowing huge bubbles, sometimes in rectangular shapes, which would shine with luminescent rainbow colors for everyone's delight.

In addition to Loon, there have been many BAC clowns at THITWGC over the years, and all of them have brought their special talents to enrich the lives of campers, staff, and volunteers. Ilene Weiss, whose clown name is Noodle, can beautifully sing everything from clown opera to improvised rap music, as well as play a variety of musical instruments. Therese Schorn, (Fidget the Clown), often wore a costume that made her look like she was riding a flamingo, whose was named Flora. As Fidget rode Flora around, the bright pink bird pecked the ground with her beak, pretending to pick up nuts. One day, the clowns announced that Flora had laid some eggs that were about to hatch. After a couple of days during which the clowns hyped up the story of Flora's eggs, Fidget and Flora proudly entered the Dining Hall followed by two campers dressed up as pink flamingo chicks.

The clowns invented other magical narratives and acts that were woven into the life of Camp and entertained us all. Fidget, thinking that a scruffy horse might be appropriate and consistent with the western theme of Camp, invented a slightly pathetic two-person horse with buckteeth and bulging eyes—and Wonky the Wonder Horse was born! Because clowns like to mythologize the ridiculous, Fidget and Loon developed the Wonky character into a hero. They devised silly emergencies to provide Wonky the opportunity to swoop in and save the day. They made grainy black and white cowboy movies featuring Wonky as the hero for campers to view, and one even included Paul. With my help as either his rear end or his trainer, Wonky often performed at the Theater and became a Camp legend.

In the early 1990s, George and Sam brought a docile Vietnamese pot-bellied pig named Betty to Camp from Green Chimneys. Betty first appeared at a carnival in front of the Dining Hall wearing a pink bow on her neck and sticking closely to Fidget's heels. Fidget and Loon would lead Betty around on a leash so that she could greet campers, wagging her tail like a dog. At one point, Betty escaped and remained on the lam for several days, with frequent pig sightings by campers and clowns. Finally, a counselor spotted Betty looking for food near the Dining Hall and recovered her so that she could again participate actively in Camp life with clowns and campers.

Staff members would frequently adopt a theme for a session. Maria Peyramaure, whose clown name is MooChacha, gave an example of clown Camp activity related to a theme:

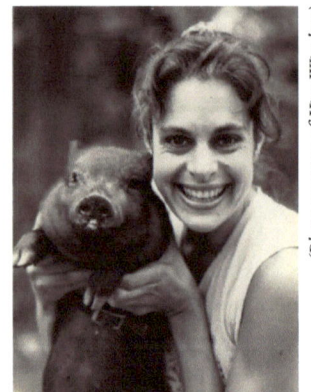

Betty with Therese/Fidget

"In my first session, the theme was along the lines of 'Weather.' We came up with a week-long treasure hunt game for the campers. The idea was that it would 'rain' something that the kids had to find; and I thought, wouldn't it be cool if it would rain 'yellow rubber duckies' on Camp? We thought of running to a few stores to try to find some ducks. But when looking for extra blankets in the basement of the Infirmary, out of the blue we found a box full of rubber duckies! My jaw dropped open! Ask and you shall receive! We spent the early mornings and rest hours strategically placing rubber duckies in random places where the campers would find them during their day activities. We announced that the cabin that found the most rubber duckies by the end of the session would receive a special prize (to 'slime' their favorite counselor, who of course, would give consent). The campers really got into the fun of finding the ducks, and each day at meals we tallied up the finds. At the end of the session, the youngest cabin Unit (seven-year-olds) had won! With the help of the very giving and generous kitchen staff, we made 'slime' with cornstarch, water, and food coloring. We laid a tarp in the center of the Dining Hall floor, placed a kiddy pool in the middle of it, and announced the winners and the prize. Everybody got to enjoy the fun of the young ones pouring green slime over their favorite counselor. Since then, I've always thought that at Camp, if you can think it, you can make it. At Camp everyone is game to create and participate in the fun, with the practice or mantra of 'Safety, Respect and Love' making it possible."

From the start, the clowns encouraged imagination, dress-up, silliness, and general theatrical creativity to cause laughter and joy among the campers. Their contribution to emotional healing is evident at each session. Over the first quarter century of Camp, well over 40 BAC clowns have participated, many coming to multiple sessions. They identify themselves with witty clown names such as Smarty Pants, Skeeter, Waffles, Quackenbush, Meatloaf, Spaghetti, and Celery Trashcan.[6] As Michael Christensen has expressed, "The positive spirit from all of the laughter and life that has manifested at Camp for so many years from so many joyful hearts is very powerful."

In addition to laughter, research has also shown that music and dancing can have a positive impact on attitudes and health through the release of tension and by encouraging self-expression

---

6 Clown list provided by Noodle/Ilene Weiss, based on an email survey of BAC clowns in the spring of 2015.

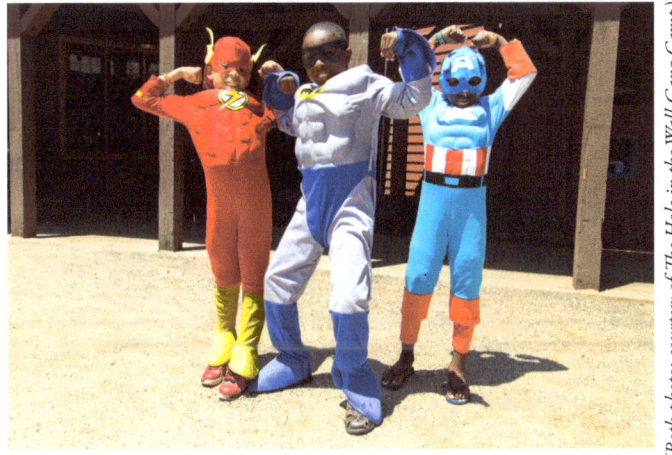
Superhero campers

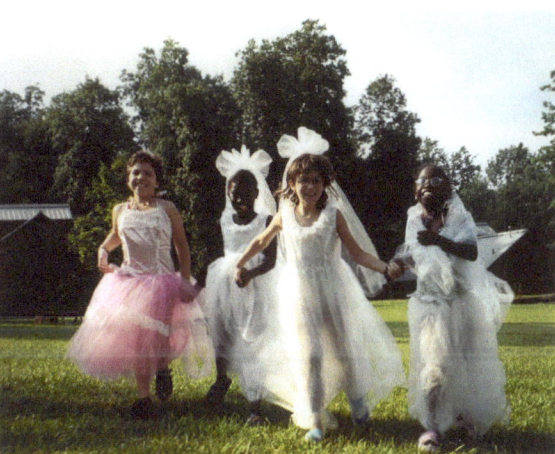
Friends in frills

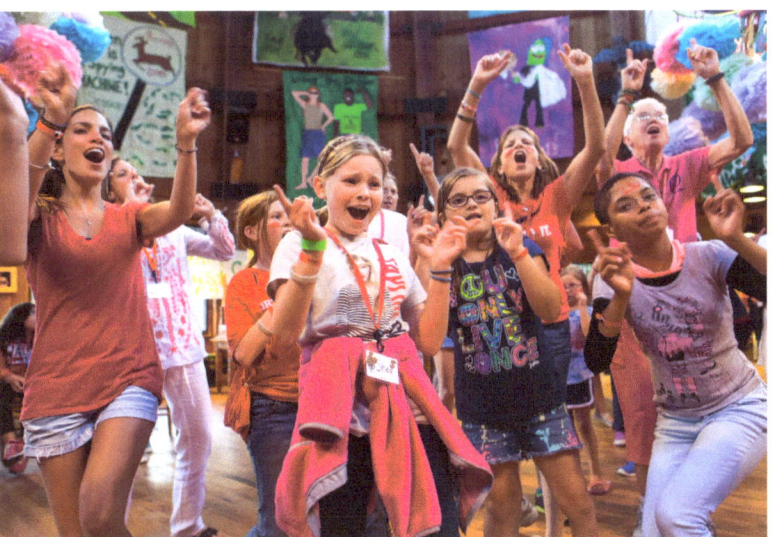
Campers shaking their bushy tails

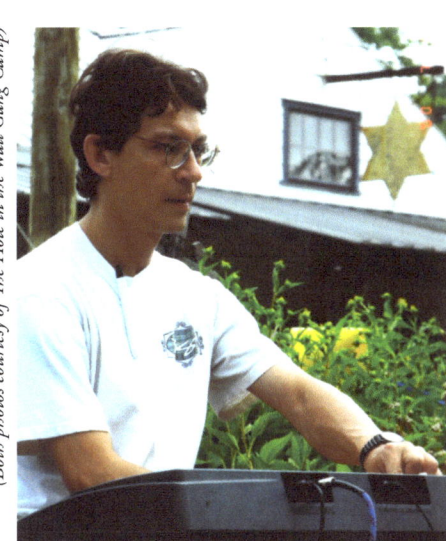
Leo at the keyboard

and a feeling of wellbeing.[7] For about 20 years, Leo Loginov-Katz filled Camp with music. Leo was born in Russia, was trained in theater, and has a gift for music. In 1989 he took a job at Samantha Smith World Peace Camp in Maine, where he directed the theater activity. This camp, opened in 1986, brings together teenagers from countries around the world where tensions and antagonisms toward others threaten peace. Israelis and Palestinians, Russians and Americans, and others have been brought to this camp to interact with each other. Leo worked at the World Peace Camp for three summers. In 1991 he facilitated the creating of a stage act by a group of Russian and American teenagers and helped them perform it. The act identified and celebrated the similarities and differences of viewpoints of the teens to help bring them together. Led by Leo, the group went

---

7   http://www.montyscorner.org/content/music-therapy-cancer?gclid=CJHn6bLesMMCFcVgf-godnJ8A2w and https://en.wikipedia.org/wiki/Dance_therapy

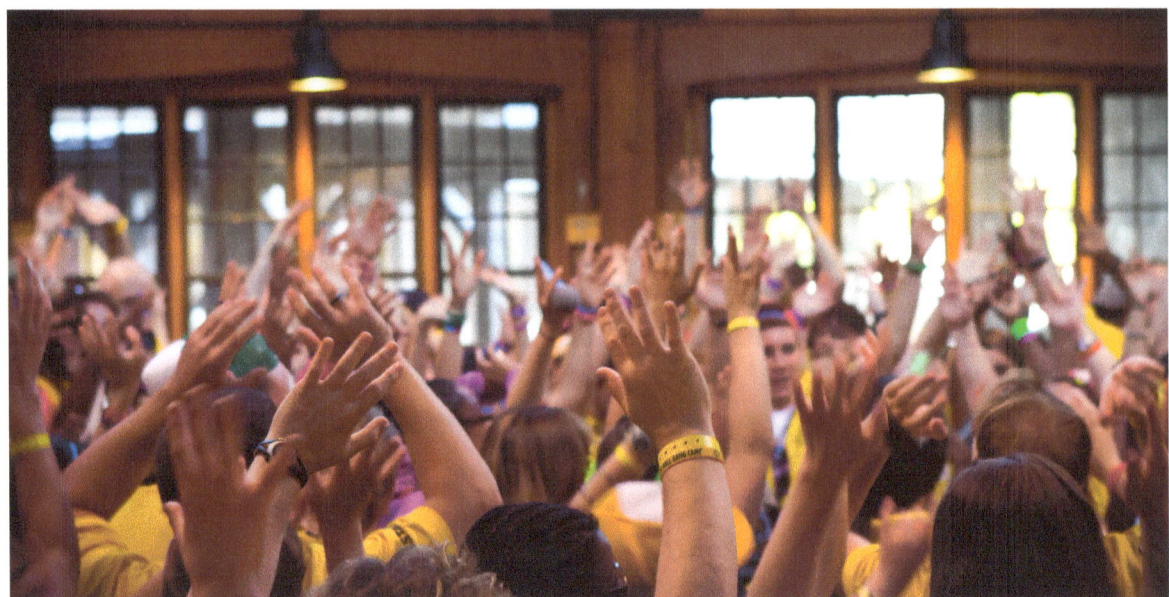

Energetic Dining Hall dancing

on the road and gave presentations throughout the Northeast, including one at the United Nations and another in THITWGC Theater. Camp Director Bob Glass was so impressed with the quality of the show that he successfully recruited Leo to join the staff and head a new theater program for campers.

Leo's first summer at THITWGC was in 1993. He integrated himself into the existing theater efforts but also began using his musical talents. He played a keyboard at mealtimes in the Dining Hall, where his fun music caused an eruption of crazy dancing in the middle of the circular eating area to songs such as "Bouncin' Round the Room." Dancing and singing after meals quickly became a tradition, with counselors and volunteers supporting campers in wheelchairs or with disabilities so that everyone could be caught up in the rhythm and joy of the moment. We all enjoyed Leo's music as we sang Camp songs such as "Camper, Camper, Shake Your Bushy Tail" and "Grandma's Feather Bed." One special song that became the unofficial Camp anthem was "Stars in the Sky." As the words of the song express, it still can "bring the summer right back to me" when I hear it.

Along with the clowns and counselors, Leo was involved in producing Stage Night, held the second from the last evening of each session. In the Theater, Leo coached and rehearsed with campers for their Stage Night acts, while Noodle and other clowns worked with the camper who would be the Master of Ceremony for the event. Campers from each Unit create and perform a skit together, and some campers give a solo performance of dancing or singing. On many occasions, Leo accompanied a young solo-

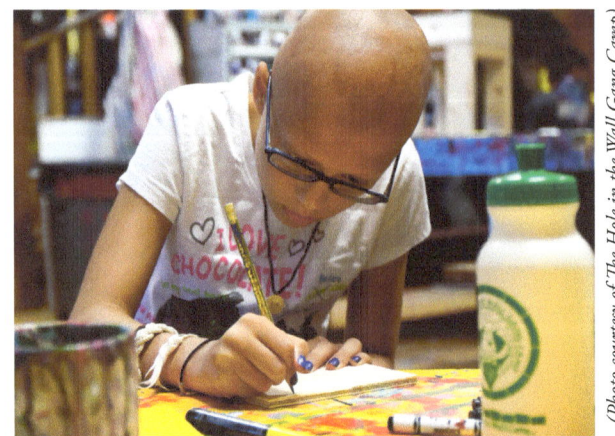

Concentrating and creating

Enthusiastic Dining Hall singing

singer whose pitch drifted during the song. Leo deftly followed the voice's pitch by changing the key of his musical accompaniment to support the singer.

On the last evening of each session, everyone meets in the Theater again for Awards Night, during which each camper receives an award for something they accomplished during the session. Volunteers are also recognized for their contributions. Music, cheering, clapping, and laughter fill the air during this event.

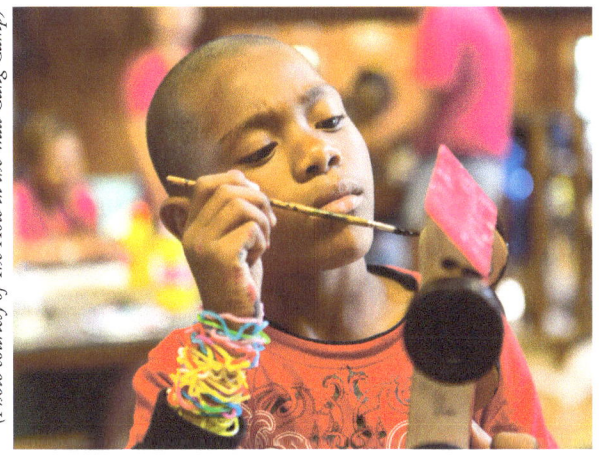

Painting in the Wood Shop

These days, every camper receives a songbook with 200 songs on arrival. The echoes of music and voices can be heard everywhere at Camp. When Noodle is on-site, she makes late evening rounds at the cabins with her ukulele-sized octave guitar for some singing with campers. Dancing is a tradition after meals but is also spontaneous at other times. Creativity is encouraged as an emotional outlet, whether in the performing arts or in Arts & Crafts. Children are often lost in deep concentration while creating something of their choice with wood, beads, ceramics, paper, or cloth. In all of the activities, we see campers living and enjoying the moment.

38 ~ CHAPTER 5 ~ Laughter, Music, Dancing, Creativity, and Emotional Healing

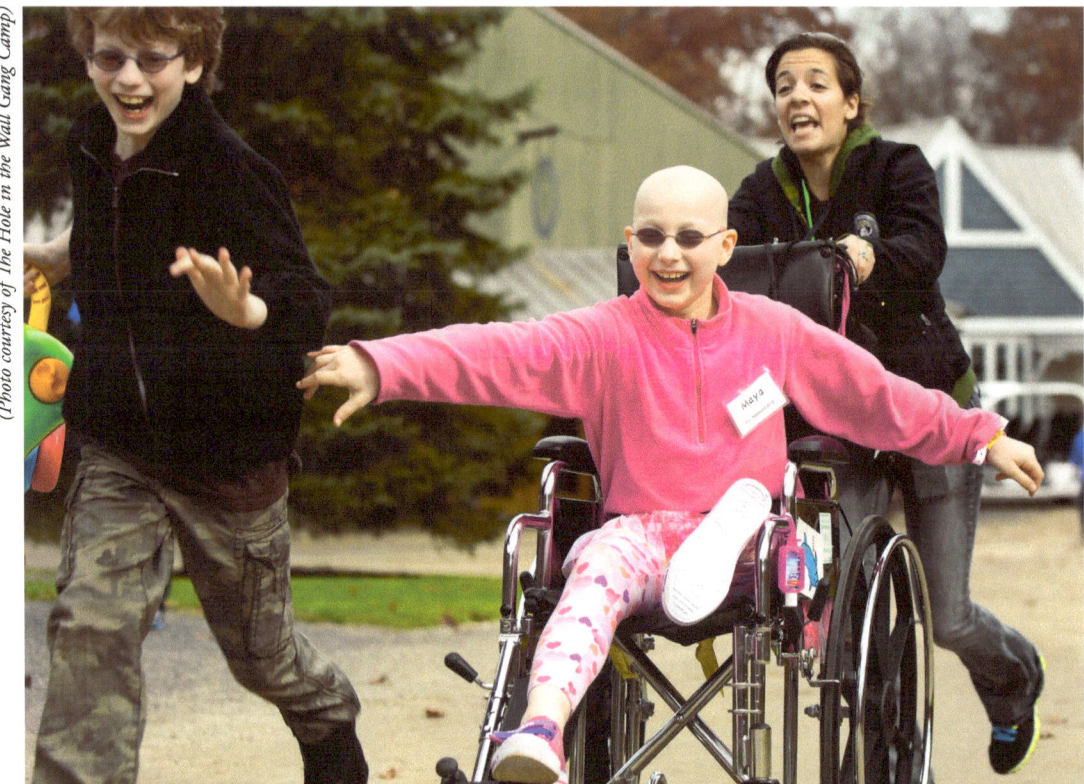
(Photo courtesy of The Hole in the Wall Gang Camp)

Enjoying the moment with exuberance

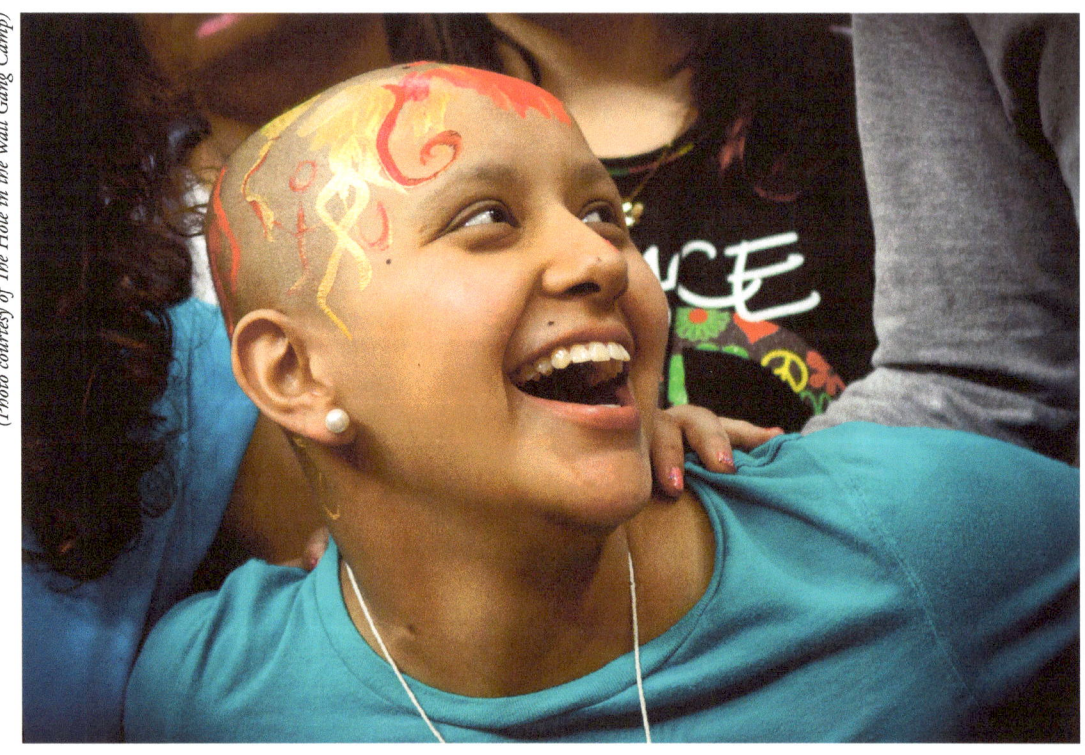
(Photo courtesy of The Hole in the Wall Gang Camp)

CHAPTER SIX

Up and Running

When Camp first opened, the medical support program was ready and waiting in the background. There was an array of activities planned by the program staff, including the Horse Barn, with gentle horses from a nearby stable; the Swimming Pool; Arts & Crafts, which included bead-working, woodworking, and other craft projects; the Gymnasium, which allowed for an array of sports and group activities; and the Boat House, where campers could fish from the dock and enjoy boating or canoeing on Pearson Pond.

Over the years, special events were added, not only in specific program areas but also Camp-wide. A scuba diving club from Providence, Rhode Island volunteered to provide campers underwater Swimming Pool adventures, including checkers games on the pool bottom. For many years, a local club provided the color of enormous hot air balloons and offered campers tethered rides with spectacular area views from the sky above the cabin circle. One year, someone brought two elephants to Camp and gave children, as well as Paul, rides on the gentle giants. Monster trucks have appeared in front of the Dining Hall. Vintage cars have driven campers around the cabin circle.

The Wood Shop allowed campers to select their projects, but building and painting a small race car quickly became a popular choice. In response, Woody and the Program Staff organized the Wood Shop 500 early on near the end of each session, creating a makeshift miniature downhill racecourse track in front of the Dining Hall for campers to "race" their cars. With lots of fanfare and hoopla from camper spectators, the children who had made race cars took turns letting their creations swoop down the course. When a car jumped off the track, a staff member would quickly put it back. At one Wood Shop 500, I saw Paul, the professional race car driver, timing each little wooden car with a stopwatch! In reality, each camper was a proud winner. Arts & Crafts had a display of camper creations at the end of each session for all to admire. Campers take home their arts and crafts to enjoy them year-round.

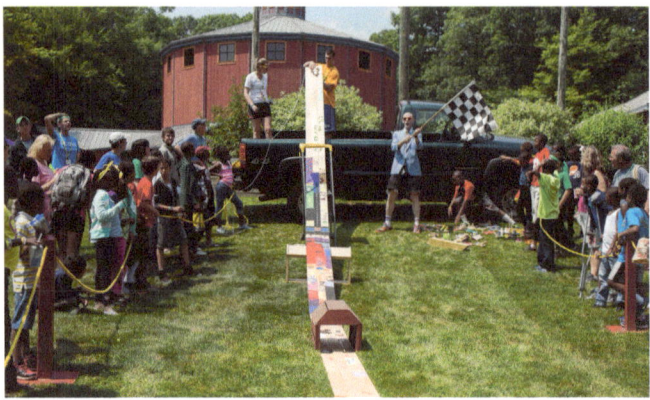
Racing at the Wood Shop 500

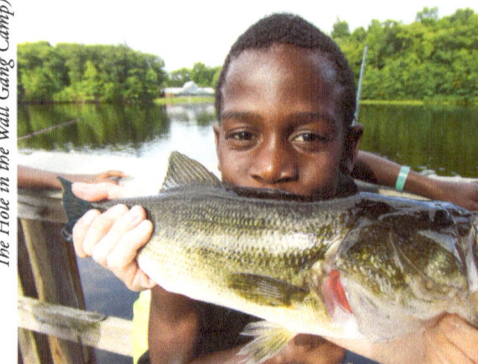
Counselor kissing a camper's catch

Traditions, legends, and special initiatives quickly started at Camp, one of which was the legend of Wee-Pee, an enormous mythical fish that lives in Pearson Pond. The name is a reverse of Peewee, which implies small in size. Wee-Pee has never been seen, but everybody wants to catch him!

Pearson Pond was stocked with bass to improve the chances of those with even the worst luck to reel in a catch. For a couple of summers during the early years, Tom Earnheart, a law professor and avid fisherman from North Carolina, was a volunteer. Tom's special initiative was "Save the Worm Week," which taught children how to make fishing flies to use instead of worms. From the beginning, campers with their counselors have fished from the pier or from a boat. There is a no-keep policy. When a fish is caught, a counselor removes the hook. It has become a tradition that the counselor kisses the fish caught by a camper before placing it back in the Pond. Part of the tradition is that campers ask, "What kind of a person kisses fish?" Their shouted answer is, "Counselors!" It is easy to identify those fish repeatedly caught by the scarring around their mouths from the hooks. Still, the beaming smiles of children holding up their catch are proof that fishing is a popular activity each session.

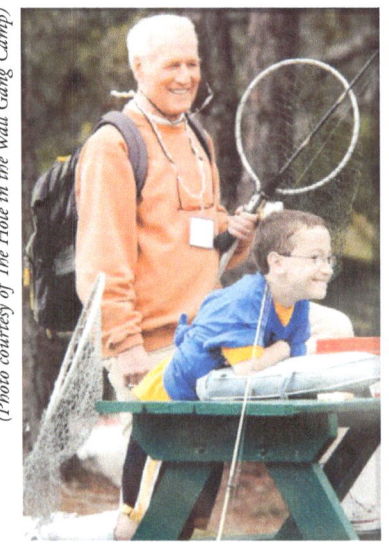
Fisherman Paul and a camper, ready to fish

Paul enjoyed fishing, but his luck was not always good. One time, a camper asked Paul, whom he did not know, to take him out on Pearson Pond to fish. Upon their return an hour later, Paul overheard the child tell a counselor, "Remind me never to go fishing with that old guy again. We didn't get a single bite!" Paul laughed uproariously.

That first summer, we had the capacity for about 90 campers, but only 40 showed up for the first session. Paul and Hotch thought that perhaps there was still great concern that families might be reluctant to send their sick children into the wilderness and away from their own doctors and hospitals. I pointed out to them that many schools in Connecticut do not end their academic year until late June, but this did not relieve their anxiety. For the rest of that first summer, we operated below capacity with 60 to 80 campers per session and had a total of only 270 individual campers for the summer. However, after the first groups of campers returned home and told their parents and doctors about their positive experiences, more and more children signed up. By the third summer, Camp was operating at capacity. The improvement in camper numbers was because of enthusiasm about the counselors, staff, friends, and the exciting summer activities. Also, we had shown families and their physicians that there was safe on-site medical and nursing coverage. We continued to have the ongoing support of the pediatric hematology/oncology community in New England.

In spite of our progress, there were still problems filling up the first sessions in June. In subsequent years, children were recruited from greater distances to fill those early sessions. Contingents of campers from Florida, Kansas City, and several European countries have participated in early June. In 1991, seven children in attendance had cancer as a result of the radioactive fallout from the meltdown in 1986 of a nuclear power plant in Chernobyl, Ukraine, which at the time was part of the Union of Soviet Socialist Republics (USSR). The fallout drifted over large parts of western USSR and Europe, causing increased rates of thyroid cancer among children. At the time, Leo was still working at the World Peace Camp in Maine, but he had visited THITWGC in 1990 on his road tour. When the Chernobyl children came to THITWGC in 1991, he provided a basic Russian-English survival language guide for the campers and counselors.

Systems at Camp, in the medical and nursing support as well as in the general activities, worked quite well beginning with the first session. As new ideas arose, they were discussed and often incorporated. The Dining Hall flow was worked out with one door for entering and the other for exiting. Mealtimes were rowdy and fun with family-styled servings at the tables. Campers stayed seated while counselors and volunteers brought food on trays and cleared the tables. The Dining Hall food quality was very high, thanks to the kitchen staff. Vegetarian meals were offered early on to those who wanted them. Newman's Own products, all donated, were ubiquitous, and today include Virgin Lemonade, Limeade, Iced Tea, cereals, coffee, and of course, salad dressing.

I think all of us involved in those first years felt a sense that we were succeeding in providing children with the experience that Paul had intended. Campers were having a great deal of fun participating in summer camp experiences that many had felt would be impossible for children with life-threatening diseases. But what was happening at The Hole in the Wall Gang Camp went beyond our expectations. Children were bonding with each other and the staff in ways that made significant progress toward emotional healing. Deep friendships were forged, along with the strong desire to return in subsequent summers that sustained children throughout the rest of the year.

After the first summer, I continued as Medical Director but also served as Executive Director in order to provide stability until the right person could be recruited to fill the position. About a year and a half later, Carroll Brewster was hired as Executive Director, which then allowed me time to campaign for and serve as President of the American Academy of Pediatrics (AAP), an organization of over 60,000 pediatricians, in 1992-1993. I continued as Medical Director and was on-site at THITWGC during the summer sessions.

We all learned that there is ample time at Camp for reflection and tears when they are needed. Emotional acceptance can be the first step toward emotional healing. The cabins were designed so that campers would have "cabin chat" opportunities for sharing and talking with each other. On one side of each cabin is the campers' bedroom, which is separated from the counselors' bedroom by a common area, originally referred to as the "dog trot." Counselors are only a shout away across the common area, but the privacy in the late evenings allowed the children to share their feelings and grow as friends.

Always in our minds were the serious illnesses of our children, and we did what we could to get them to Camp and keep them there for a full session. We heard that the doctors of one young girl from California who had been a camper did not think that she would survive until the next summer season. When Paul heard this, he visited her in California. She adamantly told him, "I will be at Camp for the first session!" Because she was unable to fly, someone provided ground transportation with drivers to bring her to Connecticut that June. She lived for that session. On the return trip to California, she became critically ill near Dallas. Her drivers called me, and I arranged for assistance at a Dallas hospital, where she was pronounced dead. We could not prevent her death, but we had enriched her life, as she enriched ours. Over the years, I have heard from numerous campers that they only lived so that they could return to Camp.

When campers grow up and "age out" of regular sessions, which are for those between seven and 15 years of age, they still want to return. THITWGC has created opportunities for this to happen. "Hero's Journey," for aged-out former campers, provides a seven-day wilderness experience during which these older adolescents learn to become "heroes of their own stories." The Leaders in Training (LIT) program, offered to older former campers, provides them with the opportunity to work with current campers and participate in leadership workshops. Many young people from the LIT program return as counselors. About 20% to 30% of our counselors today were previous campers, and they often remark how important it is for them to give something back to Camp.

Much has been told about the positive influence of THITWGC on children, but Camp has also had major influences on the lives and careers of the counselors and staff. One example of a staff member who changed his career direction because of Camp is Nick Evageliou. In 1990, Nick was an undergraduate at the University of Maryland majoring in political science when he responded to a posting for a summer job as a driver for THITWGC. Nick was hired and spent the summer interacting with staff and the children. He was so impressed with the people and the place that he returned the following two summers as a counselor. As his interest in the medical aspects of Camp grew, Nick spent time observing in the Infirmary and had a number of evening discussions with me about medicine. After his graduation from Maryland, he entered the Tufts University graduate program in international relations, aiming for a career in the Foreign Service. But when he realized that he found medicine much more compelling, Nick submitted applications to medical schools. The essay in his applications described that his interest in medicine was in large part because of his experience at THITWGC.

The next year Nick entered the University of Connecticut Medical School. After graduation, he did his pediatric residency at Children's Hospital of Philadelphia (CHOP), followed by a fellowship in pediatric hematology/oncology at the same institution. He then joined the pediatric faculty of the University of Pennsylvania School of Medicine, where he is today, treating patients with cancer and blood disorders and doing research on Wilms' tumor. In the summer of 2014, Nick returned to THITWGC as a volunteer physician along with his wife, who is a pediatric cardiologist. Nick's mother, who lives near Camp, still visits during each session to help campers dressing up in their costumes for Stage Night.

Matt Burke also chose a career in medicine after being involved with Camp for many years. Matt was diagnosed with acute lymphoblastic leukemia when he was nine years old. He was essentially forced to attend in 1989 by his mother, who saw a *LIFE* magazine article about THITWGC while in a hospital waiting room during one of Matt's radiation treatments. In contrast to Nick, Matt did not like his first year's experience—he suffered from homesickness and failed to make friends. But when his parents forced him to return again the following summer, everything fell into place for him. He was assigned to Jimmy Canton's cabin and immediately bonded with other campers. (Jimmy has worked at THITWGC since it opened and now in 2016 is the Chief Executive Officer.) Matt enthusiastically returned as a camper each summer through 1995 and then attended as an LIT. He was subsequently on the staff for three years. He identifies THITWGC as being different from other summer camps because of its "heart and energy." On Matt's application to medical school, he wrote, "My counselors are the kind of people that I really want to become in terms of the way they deal with people and treat people." Matt has reflected eloquently on the emotional and physical healing that occurs:

"I've seen kids survive well beyond their doctors' expectations in order to get back to Camp. A prognosis of a couple months turns into a year, so they can come back another summer. I've seen kids who have zero blood counts come to Camp against their doctors' orders, and their health just bloomed. I remember a child who came to Camp who was very frail. She actually lasted the whole session and got stronger at Camp. She died two days after leaving Camp."

Matt became a family practice physician. He is currently on the faculty of the Department of Family Medicine at Franklin Square Medical Center in Baltimore, Maryland. He serves on the board of the Maryland Academy of Family Physicians and is an assistant professor in family medicine at Georgetown University.

THITWGC also was a guiding influence in the career path that my granddaughter Jennifer (Jen) chose. She lived with Anne and me when she was growing up, and she closely followed the development of Camp from the beginning. Jen became a trained equestrienne and spent part of the summer of 1998 working in the Horse Barn. She returned full-time in 1999 as the equine Program Specialist and subsequently volunteered in that capacity in 2000 and 2001. During those years, she was encouraged by a number of social workers who had accompanied children to Camp to consider social work as a profession because of its opportunities to utilize alternative therapies, including therapeutic riding and animal-assisted therapy (AAT). At that time, AAT was just beginning to gain popularity, and Jen often visited Dr. Sam Ross at Green Chimneys to learn more about the field. She went on to earn a Master of Social Work (MSW) with a specialization in AAT from the University of Denver and a Master of Science (MS) in Applied Animal Behaviour and Animal Welfare from the University of Edinburgh in Scotland. Jen has been on the faculty of the University of Denver's Institute for Human-Animal Connection since 2008 and is currently pursuing a doctorate in human-animal interactions there. She lectures internationally on AAT and the welfare of therapy animals.

Nick, Matt, and Jen are only three examples of alumni whose lives changed because of the positive and healing atmosphere of THITWGC centered on laughter, music, dancing, fun, and

CHAPTER 6 ~ Up and Running

creativity. Many campers and staff keep in touch with each other long after the summer is over. Some campers give directly back to Camp by returning as staff or volunteers. Present campers are reassured and inspired by the interactions with those who have faced and beaten their own serious illnesses.

Early in the planning for THITWGC, I knew that the support of the region's pediatric medical community was essential for camper recruitment and long-term success. Active involvement by medical providers soon became routine during the summer. While some medical people visited only for a day, many became regular volunteers. My pediatric hematology/oncology fellows from Yale came up for a session each summer. I combined volunteering and learning opportunities for medical students and residents by offering electives in pediatric hematology/oncology. A significant medical volunteer from my personal perspective was my son Stephen, a general pediatrician who has spent his career in community health centers serving the children of migrant and seasonal farm workers in the Pacific Northwest. Stephen volunteered for a session during each of three different years.

Other physicians who have been long-term volunteers at Camp are listed here:

- Dr. Eileen Gillan, a pediatric hematologist/oncologist from the University of Connecticut Medical School and Connecticut Children's Medical Center in Hartford (CCMC), succeeded me as Medical Director for two years. However, she was also a member of the U.S. Army Reserve and was called up for duty in Iraq. (At that point, Dr. Sharon Space became THITWGC Medical Director.) As of 2014, Eileen had volunteered at Camp for 20 years.
- Dr. Dave Nelson began volunteering when he was a fellow in pediatric emergency medicine in Rhode Island. He has continued volunteering since he moved to Las Vegas years ago and currently tallies 15 years at Camp.
- Dr. Jenny Schwab, a general pediatrician in Rocky Hill, Connecticut, has 14 continuous years as a volunteer, beginning when she was a pediatric resident at CCMC.
- Dr. Molly Schwenn, a pediatric hematologist/oncologist, volunteered a session each year for 12 summers, from 1990 to 2001, when she moved to Maine.
- Dr. Lorna Seybolt has volunteered for the past 12 years at all of the Immunology Sessions (described later). She first volunteered when she was a pediatric infectious disease fellow at Boston Medical Center. Moving out of the area, first to Maine and then to New Orleans, has

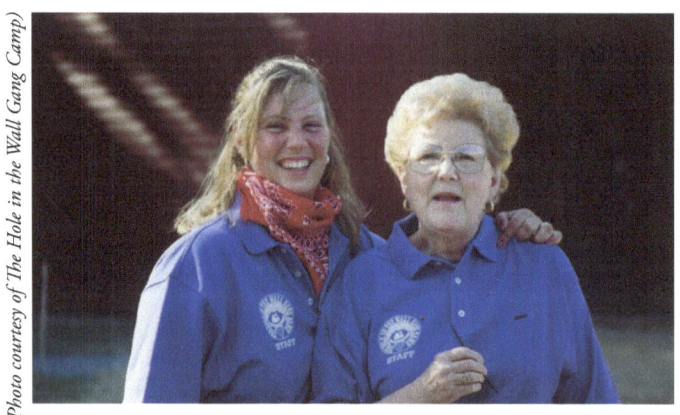

(Photo courtesy of The Hole in the Wall Gang Camp)

Jen and my wife Anne at Camp

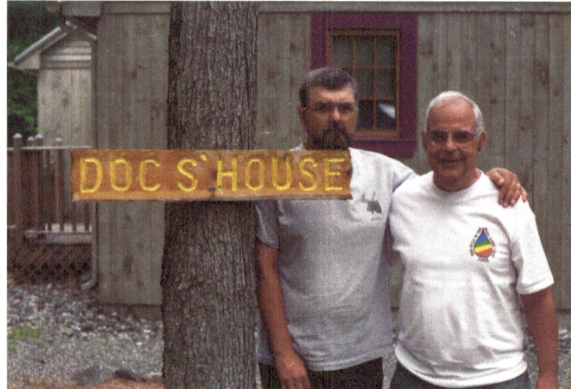

With my son Stephen at Doc's House

not interrupted her volunteering at Camp. She also serves on our Medical Committee.
- Dr. Matt Heeney, Professor of Pediatrics and head of the Sickle Cell Service at Boston Children's Hospital, currently has 11 years as a volunteer. He brings about 40 children from his medical service to a Sickle Cell Session (described later) each summer.
- Dr. Kerry Moss began volunteering when she was a CCMC Pediatric resident ten years ago. Now she volunteers at Camp as a CCMC pediatric hematologist/oncologist.

During my tenure and Sue's, there were a number of nurses who served as staff members and volunteers for multiple years including Maureen Gallagher, Sara Bodenmiller, Joanie Morris (nee Krise), Emily Sadinski, Tad Dorry, Jeanine Lutz, and Joyce Simpson. In any given year, total volunteers can number in the hundreds. In 2010, there were over 60 medical and nursing volunteers and over 400 non-medical volunteers.[1]

There are many more who have given their time and energy to make THITWGC the safe and healing place that it is. They have commented on the powerful, exceptional experience Camp provides to campers as well as volunteers. One of my Yale pediatric hematology/oncology fellows, Dr. Cliff Selsky, who came several summers, commented to me on the last day of his first session as a volunteer, "Well, I'm going back to New Haven, back to the real world." I replied, "No, this is real world." For the children, staff, and volunteers alike, Camp becomes our real, healing world each summer.

---

1   http://www.holeinthewallgang.org/Customer-Content/www/News/PDFs/Gazettes/Gazette-2011-Fall.pdf

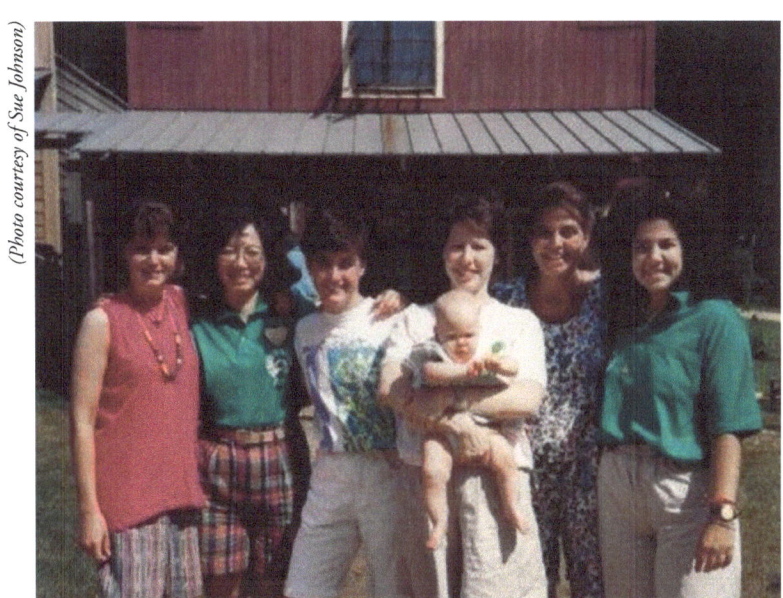

Nursing staff in 1992. Left to right:
Sara Bodenmiller, RN; Vita Goei, MD (volunteer); Joanie Krise, RN;
Sue Staples Johnson, APRN (with daughter Sara);
Donna Nucci, RN (volunteer); Nancy Maloney, RN (volunteer).

CHAPTER SEVEN

Celebrities

Paul Newman's celebrity has been an enormous help to THITWGC throughout its existence. He was easily recognized, in spite of the fact that he wore dark sunglasses most of the time he was in public to cover his blue eyes. One day when he was in New Haven, he suggested that we have lunch at a restaurant. Paul was dressed in a sweat suit without pockets (and no money) because he was going to work out. As usual, he had on large dark sunglasses and commented to me that he preferred to be incognito in public. After Paul had excused himself to the restroom, the headwaiter came over and asked, "Is that who I think it is?" So much for incognito! After the meal, I gave my credit card to the waitress. When she returned with the tab, I signed it. She commented, "Oh, &#!!, I wanted HIS autograph!"

While Paul was a very private person who shied away from signing autographs in public, he always obliged a camper who asked for his autograph, even if it was for someone else. He spent as much time at Camp as his movie-making schedule would allow—during the first couple of years he was present for two to four days almost every session. He ate with the children in the Dining Hall, browsed through the Wood Shop to admire the race cars campers were making, and took campers fishing. To facilitate and perhaps prolong his visits, he built a cabin on a quiet, private shore of Pearson Pond. He and Joanne were often seen riding around Camp on their bicycles.

On one occasion, Paul was in the Dining Hall eating with the children when he noticed a child looking intently at him and then at his picture on a carton of Newman's Own Virgin Lemonade on the table. Paul finally asked him, "Don't you know who that is?" The camper retorted, "Geeze, mister, were you missing?" During one Sickle Cell Special Session, Paul was a volunteer counselor for one of the boys' Units. Although he stayed in his own cabin at night, he bicycled to the Unit early each morning and spent all day with the campers. At the end of that session, the children clung to Paul, not wanting to let go and get on the bus that would take them away from Camp. Tears were shed, although Paul tried to hide his behind sunglasses.

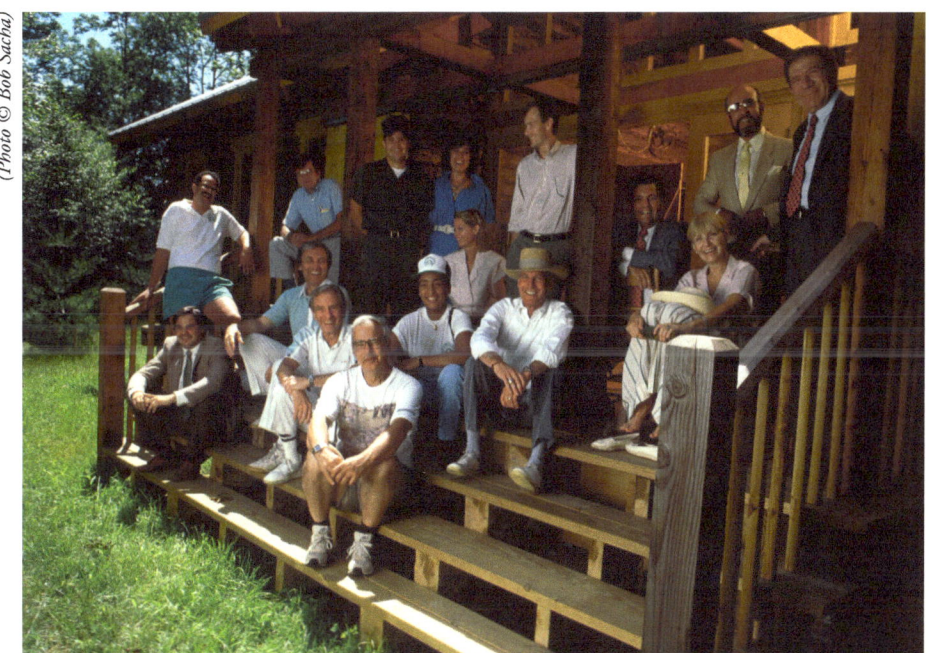

Original Board members and others on a cabin porch, 1988 – From LIFE magazine. Sitting (L to R): Mike Kolakowski, Ray Lamontagne, A.E. Hotchner, Doc Pearson, Ursula Hotchner, Paul Newman, Kahled Alhegelan, Joanne Woodward. Standing: Jeff Glick, unidentified, a Seabee Volunteer, Shivaun Manley, unidentified, Vince Conti, unidentified, Simon Konover.

During the summer of 1988, *LIFE* magazine approached Paul about covering the story of THITWGC. He agreed but insisted that the emphasis be on the Board members and other people who helped make Camp happen rather than on him. What resulted was the September 1, 1988 edition of *LIFE* with a picture of Paul and some campers as well as "Paul Newman's Dream" in bold black letters on the cover. Although there was a nice photograph of some of the original Board and other people, Paul felt that the magazine cover and article did not appropriately reflect his request. Nonetheless, I do know that the publicity we received prompted some families to allow their children (including Matt Burke) to become campers. It also facilitated recruitment of staff and volunteers from all over the country. Over the years, Paul persistently resisted publicity for Camp because he did not want it to end up being about him. I have been told by a number of people that THITWGC is one of the best-kept secrets in Connecticut.

Throughout the years, the Board has continued to evolve and has included individuals who are celebrities in my mind. Khaled Alhegelan and Ray Lamontagne still serve, as do Ursula (whose last name is now Gwynne) and Hotch. Paul's daughter Melissa (Lissy) is an active Board member and Camp volunteer. At my suggestion, Karen Hendricks, J.D., joined the Board, becoming its first African-American member. She had worked as my legislative advisor in Washington, D.C., while I served as President of the American Academy of Pediatrics. Karen's advocacy for children in general grew to include our campers. She served on the Board until the autumn of 2015.

Paul's celebrity connections have attracted a few Board members as well as Camp volunteers from among the nationally famous. The most effective celebrities have been those who set aside their own egos or personae and, as volunteers, focus on the needs of the campers. As a baseball fan, I was pleased when Sandy Koufax of the Los Angeles Dodgers joined the Board. Sandy, one of baseball's greatest pitchers of all time, had four no-hitters (including one perfect game), three Cy Young Awards, and was the youngest player ever elected to the Baseball Hall of Fame.[1] As a Board member, his focus is on the children, although he expressed disappointment in me at Camp's 25th birthday party when I told him that I am a Boston Red Sox fan.

Another celebrity who volunteered as a counselor during a very hot and sultry session in 2001 was called "Jules" by the staff at her request. During that session, I had my pediatrician son Stephen volunteering with me, while his wife Mary Lou (my co-author) volunteered wherever she was needed. One morning, Mary Lou was assigned to help out in the Horse Barn with some of the youngest campers. Jules, an attractive woman wearing overalls and a bandanna over her pigtailed hair was with that Unit. The riding activities proceeded in the stifling heat of the Horse Barn. At lunch when Mary Lou related her morning activity to me, I asked her how Jules was doing. She replied, "Oh, she's sweating along with the rest of us!" Later that evening, Paul arrived for a visit, and one of the first things he asked me was, "How is she doing?" Knowing immediately who "she" was, I replied, "Oh, she's sweating along with the rest of us!" I indicated that she was giving 100% to the children. Paul was delighted with that response. Jules was staying in the cabins (not air conditioned at that time), did not waste time putting on makeup, and clearly loved the experience. Sue related to me that she was helping staff at the top of the Tower one afternoon when Jules attempted to climb it. She seemed terrified during the ascent. When she reached the top, shaking from the experience, she enthusiastically hugged Sue and told her that she had wanted to set a good example for the campers by climbing. Jules then sped down the zip line. When the session ended, a stretch limousine pulled up to the Administration building to wait for Jules, who was transforming herself with elegant clothing, hairdo, and cosmetics back to the actress Julia Roberts, who became a member of the Board.

Actor, film producer, and comedian Alec Baldwin joined the Board and has made numerous visits to Camp. Actor and director James (Jim) Naughton, a graduate of the Yale Drama School, is also active as a Board member and in the production of recent Galas. Actor, movie director, and producer Bradley Cooper has been a volunteer counselor and currently serves on the Board.

The celebrity participation is overtly seen during the Camp Galas that are organized on a yearly basis to raise funds. Because families and children participate in Camp programs without any cost to them, there is a continuous, ongoing effort to raise money to sustain all of the activities. The idea for the Gala originally came from Hotch. Once the Theater was built, he suggested to Paul that we should have an on site fundraising event with celebrities. Paul was dubious that celebrities would come three hours from New York City to perform and also that an audience could be attracted, but he was willing to give it a try. Years later, Hotch described the first Gala that took place in September 1990:

> "I asked 15 celebrities to come to Ashford and perform with the children. I thought that maybe a couple of them would come, but what happened was that all 15 accepted…I had these wonderful artists coming from New York to perform, and I had to tell them, 'Do you

---

1   http://en.wikipedia.org/wiki/Sandy_Koufax

mind if you do just do one song?' But they were great about it. After this experience, I reduced the number of celebrities invited. But we have had an influx of celebrity performers at the Galas over the years, everyone from Cy Colman to Julia Roberts to Alec Baldwin to Whoopi Goldberg to Jim Naughton, etc., etc., -- a virtual Who's Who of the entertainment business. Newman performed every year and was a good sport…[sometimes he was] in drag, [and one year] I had him play Tinker Bell. The celebrities performed with a group of campers."

The Galas generally were staged in September, when sessions were over for the year but Camp was at its most beautiful because of the autumn foliage. All 280 seats were sold, which when combined with a silent auction, resulted in significant financial donations to Camp. Hotch commented about the Galas in general, "For me the greatest gratification is the delight and joyfulness of the children who have been granted the privilege of performing with these generous stars. It is something that will stay with them long afterward."

In 2008, the Gala was moved to New York City to increase the fundraising potential. It was Paul's last Gala. On March 10th of that year, it was held in the New York City Center in celebration of Camp's 20th anniversary. The three-hour program, written and staged by Hotch, included 15 celebrities and 25 campers. A take-off from *The Wizard of Oz* was included, featuring Joanne Woodward as the Wicked Witch of the West and Paul as the Cowardly Lion. That Gala pushed the amount raised through these events over the $15,000,000 mark. Celebrities and campers had played before audiences totaling over 6,000 people. Five years later in 2013, the Gala was held at the Lincoln Center in New York City. Jim Naughton staged and produced the program, which marked the 25th anniversary of THITWGC. One of the most poignant moments was the performance of camper Maggie, who danced with grace on her prosthesis.

Although Paul is no longer with us, his daughter and Board member Lissy has been a summer volunteer since 2009. When talking about the magic of Camp, Lissy described "the utter joy, laughter, and downright nuttiness there."

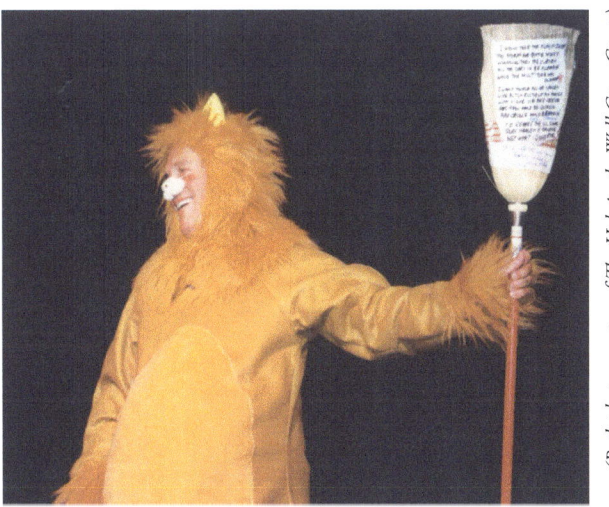

Paul as the Cowardly Lion from The Wizard of Oz, 2008

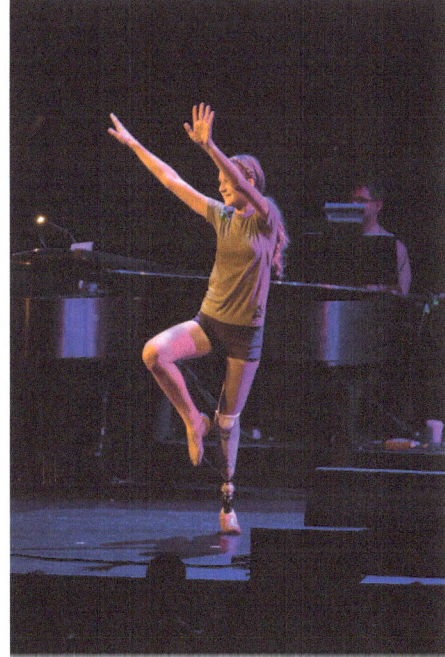

(Both photos courtesy of The Hole in the Wall Gang Camp)

Maggie dancing at the Lincoln Center Gala, 2013

CHAPTER EIGHT

Diseases of the Children at Camp

"I remember when during our first session in 1991, a 14-year-old kid who was sitting next to me at lunch told me that this was his third summer at Camp. He had a brain tumor and had several very serious operations. These saved his life, but he developed seizures and severe headaches. He said that his life was nothing but one headache followed by another headache—on and on—until he comes to Camp. I can't think of anything more eloquent than what he had to say." - Paul Newman

The Hole in the Wall Gang Camp was designed to be handicapped-accessible, and the medical program was planned to be non-intrusive but medically safe for the children. Beyond the physical aspects of any medically related camp, the most important decisions are determining which children will be served, the extent of their illnesses, and what medical support services are needed for them in transit and on site. Many children at Camp are still receiving chemotherapy. Over the years, our highest priority has been to accept children who, because of their diseases and their complications or treatment, would most benefit from Camp. Almost all of the campers during our first few years had cancer or serious blood diseases, and many of them came from the pediatric hematology/oncology clinics at Yale and the University of Connecticut. There are now nine sessions each summer lasting seven days, with approximately 120 children at each session and a staff/volunteer to child ratio of 1:2. Overall, the general attitude or approach for interacting with children during a session is that they are kids who ought to be allowed to have fun. Although their bodies may have life-threatening diseases, they are first and foremost children.

During almost every session, I held a "Doc's Chat" for volunteers and staff to inform them about Camp, the diseases, and the realities of what we were doing as well as to allow them to ask me questions. On a few occasions, when a child passed away shortly after leaving Camp as Philip had the first year, some of the counselors expressed concern that perhaps the activities at Camp had hastened the death. I reassured them that death occurred because we accepted children who were very ill. Understanding the campers' diseases described below should give insight into the challenges at THITWGC. Although I use medical terminology, I explain technical words for non-medical people.

Cancers

In fulfillment of Paul's original dream of a camp for children with cancer, many of our campers have a cancer diagnosis. From the start, we anticipated their medical needs and devised creative ways to address them so that the children can experience Camp to the fullest. Childhood cancers are very different from cancer in adults. The cancers that are most prevalent in adults—breast, lung, prostate, stomach, and colonic—rarely, if ever, occur in children. Children most commonly have leukemia (cancer of the blood), followed closely by brain cancer. Additional types of cancer seen in children and adolescents include lymphoma (cancer of the lymph glands), and a variety of solid tumors involving the bones, muscles, or internal organs such as the kidney. Pediatric cancers are treated with various combinations of chemotherapy, surgery, and radiation therapy, depending on the type of cancer. Overall in the United States from 2004 to 2010, 83% of children ages 0 to 14 years diagnosed with cancer survived. This is an improvement from 1975 to 1977, when only 58% of children with cancer survived.[1]

There are usually ten or more children with internal ports during an average general session at Camp. A port is inserted into a child's arm during cancer treatment to deliver multiple blood and platelet transfusions necessary for treatment of the disease as well as to deal with the toxic effects of some medications. A closed or internal port involves surgically inserting a plastic reservoir connected to a deep vein under the skin. A needle can then be inserted through the skin into the port to give medications or transfusions or to obtain blood for testing. Some children receiving more intensive and frequent treatments have external ports or "broviacs," which are inserted into a large vein through the chest wall. These are usually used during the initial stages of treatment. Rather than connecting to a reservoir under the skin as in an internal port, these tubes are connected to a deep vein and come out of the chest wall. Broviacs are easier on both medical personnel and children because they avoid frequent needle sticks for medicine administration and blood draws. To avoid infection, they need special care daily, including sterile dressings. In most general sessions at Camp, there are three or four children with broviacs. In our first few summers, we did not permit children with broviacs to go swimming. However, we learned that when an external port is covered with a special bandage in the Infirmary just before going to the pool and then cleaned and dressed in the Infirmary immediately afterwards, the

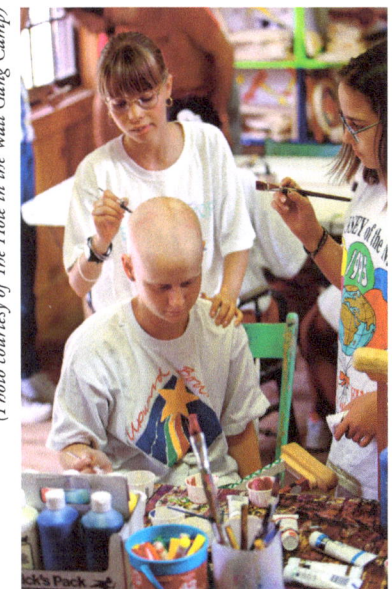

Camper having a peace sign painted on her bald head

(Photo courtesy of The Hole in the Wall Gang Camp)

---

1 Childhood Cancer–Cancer Statistics Review, Table 28.8, National Cancer Institute, 2014 <http://seer.cancer.gov/csr/1975_2011/results_merged/sect_28_childhood_cancer.pdf>.

risk of infection does not increase. Children with broviacs can now go into the pool and enjoy swimming if we have their doctor's permission.

Leukemia (blood cancer) is the most common pediatric cancer in the population at large as well as at THITWGC. The most prevalent type of childhood leukemia is acute lymphoblastic leukemia (ALL). Treatment consists of chemotherapy over a two- to three-year period. Hair loss is common during the first phases of treatment. At Camp, hair loss is destigmatized by children putting their wigs and hats aside and perhaps having their bald heads painted in Arts & Crafts. Sometimes their counselors shave their own heads.

When I began medical school in the 1950s, ALL was almost always a fatal disease, with survival of only a few months. By 2010, a substantial number of drugs and treatment protocols had been developed that resulted in a cure rate of 92% in children with ALL.[2] Treatment starts with systemic chemotherapy to kill as many of the leukemic cells as possible. This first stage of treatment is called "induction" and produces a remission in almost all children, with a return to normal blood counts and an eradication of ALL cancer cells from the blood and bone marrow. If nothing else is done, the leukemia is likely to recur. Consequently, more aggressive chemotherapy is used for several months, called "consolidation," which includes injections of chemotherapy into the spinal fluid to treat leukemic cells in "sanctuaries" in the brain that are not reached by systemic chemotherapy.

After the consolidation stage, the children are placed into "maintenance therapy," during which they receive oral medications as well as periodic injections. Maintenance therapy usually lasts for two years. Camp sessions have many children on maintenance therapy for ALL and also children who are in long-term remission and considered to be cured. If a child has gone a period of three years without a relapse (a return of the leukemia process), the likelihood of recurrence is very small. This has been a major medical triumph!

Unfortunately, some children with ALL do relapse. When that happens, some of them may receive a bone marrow transplant in an attempt to increase the chance of long-term survival/cure. But every year we hear that a few campers from previous summers have died.

There are other types of leukemia, including acute myelogenous leukemia (AML), the next most common form of the disease. AML is treated differently than ALL, and the treatment is more difficult with less successful outcomes. In 2010, only 66% of children aged 0 to 14 with AML had a five-year or more survival rate.[3]

Children with a leukemia diagnosis usually come to Camp when they are comfortably into the maintenance therapy stage, but occasionally we have a child who is still weak and debilitated during the consolidation stage. One such child was a frail seven-year-old boy not yet able to walk again. Pale and bald from the chemotherapy, this camper was transported by golf cart and on the back of Camp Director Bob Glass. As the more mobile campers of his Unit walked the pathways from one activity to the next, Bob shuttled his camper along with the others. Throughout the session, the boy was integrated into all of his Unit's activities, including Stage Night when he and Bob were on the Theater's stage with the group, singing and having fun. During the course of the session, the camper's pale face showed increasing color, and his eyes reflected the joy of being at Camp.

---

2   *ibid.*
3   *ibid.*

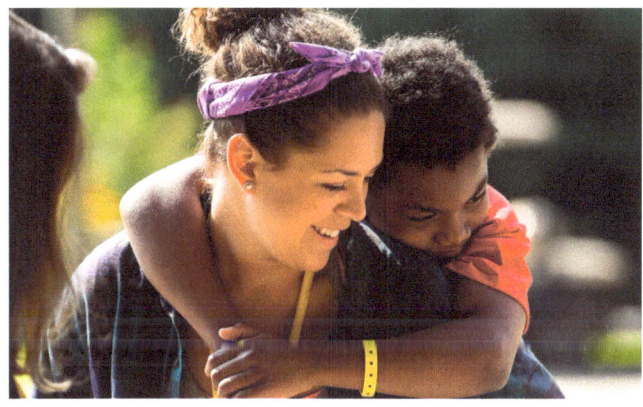
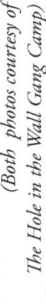

Camper on a counselor's back *Using crutches as microphones in the Dining Hall*

(Both photos courtesy of The Hole in the Wall Gang Camp)

Brain tumors account for the next most common pediatric cancers. There are different types of brain tumors, such as glioblastoma, pituitary, meduloblastoma, and ependymoma. Treatment varies based on the tumor type and its location; and it can include surgery, radiation, and chemotherapy. In most cases, the first line of therapy is surgery to remove as much of the tumor as possible. This is often followed by radiation therapy to treat any residual tumor. The survival rate of children with brain cancer has markedly improved over the years, and today it is approximately 75%, depending on the type of tumor. Despite these improved survival rates, many of these children have long-term neurological consequences from the primary disease as well as its treatments. Many children cured of brain cancer have learning disabilities as well as endocrine, growth, and developmental problems. Living with these children at Camp, I have seen them trying bravely to cope with and adapt to the long-term consequences.

Mobility is a common challenge for children with brain cancer and other malignancies. At THITWGC, in addition to having a fleet of golf carts for use as needed, staff and volunteers pitch in to get campers where they need or want to go. Sometimes counselors transport campers on their backs. Mary Lou recalls a camper, unable to walk due to brain cancer surgery, participating in the Ropes Challenge Course with her Unit one morning. The golf cart took the ten-year-old to within 20 yards of the Course. Too large for a ride on someone's back, the camper made it the rest of the way to the site supported by Mary Lou walking behind her with arms under the camper's armpits. Once at the Course, the camper was able to join in with cheers and shouts of joy as the Unit's campers collaboratively met the challenges of the Course. Mary Lou returned her camper to the golf cart by means of the same supportive walk.

Lymphomas are malignancies involving the lymph glands. There are two types of lymphoma: Hodgkin's disease and non-Hodgkin's lymphoma. Children with lymphoma usually present with enlarged lymph nodes in the neck, chest, or abdomen and sometimes with an enlarged spleen. The treatment includes intensive chemotherapy and sometimes radiation therapy. Thirty years ago, Hodgkin's disease was almost always fatal. Today, about 95% of children will be cured by one to two years of aggressive treatment. The cure rate for non-Hodgkin's lymphoma is not quite as high (about 80%) because it tends to spread widely.

THITWGC serves children with a variety of solid tumors involving internal organs or tissues. Neuroblastoma is a cancer of the sympathetic nervous tissue, often found in the adrenal glands. It is treated with a combination of chemotherapy, surgery, and, in advanced cases, stem cell transplant. Survival rates vary greatly depending on the age, specific diagnosis, and site of the tumor. In general, younger children with small tumors have higher survival rates. Wilms' tumor is cancer of the kidney. Removal of the affected kidney, followed by chemotherapy and sometimes radiation, will result in 90% cure rates. Osteosarcoma is bone cancer. Treatment is primarily surgery and chemotherapy, with radiation sometimes used as well. Ewing sarcoma, a cancerous tumor in

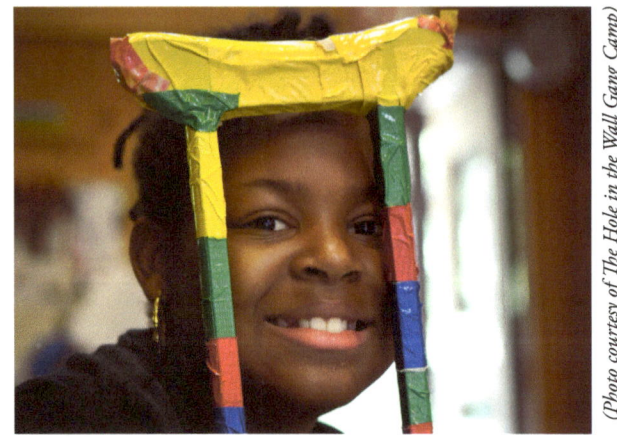

Camper with crutches decorated by Sherry

the bone or in the soft tissue around bone, is treated with chemotherapy and sometimes surgery. The children with osteosarcoma or Ewing sarcoma can have a limp or amputation, and they might need crutches or wheelchairs to get around. At Camp, our mural painter Sherry has helped children decorate their crutches in Arts and Crafts. At Yale-New Haven Hospital several years ago, two children who did not know each other recognized that they had both been campers because of their colorful crutches.

When I began my specialty career in pediatric hematology/oncology over a half-century ago, bone tumors were almost always fatal. Now the cure rate is about 70%. Rhabdomyosarcoma, muscle cancer, is treated with surgery, chemotherapy, and radiation therapy. Survival rates vary from 50% to 65%, depending on the child's age and site of the tumor.

Blood Diseases

Hemophilia is a genetic bleeding disease that results from abnormal genes located on the X chromosome so it almost exclusively affects males. Boys with hemophilia have very low levels of specific clotting factors. The Centers for Disease Control and Prevention estimates that there are approximately 20,000 hemophilia patients in the United States, and that about one in 5,000 males born has the disease.[4] There are two major forms of hemophilia: Classical Hemophilia (or Hemophilia A) and Hemophilia B (also called Christmas Disease). In Hemophilia A, the body does not adequately produce clotting Factor VIII (anti-hemophilic globulin or AHG). In Hemophilia B, clotting Factor IX is not produced adequately. About 80% of hemophiliac boys have Hemophilia A, and 20% have Hemophilia B. These Factors are necessary for normal clotting of the blood. Because of a deficiency of these clotting factors, the boys often experience bleeding into their large joints—shoulders, hips, knees, or ankles—with even a minor injury or spontaneously in the absence of an injury, which can result in severe pain, inflammation, or damage to the joint. Injections of the concentrated preparations of the missing Factor are effective in stopping the bleeding, but they must be given intravenously and often repeatedly. Boys with hemophilia bring

---

4 Centers for Disease Control and Prevention, Hemophilia, Data and Statistics, 2014 <http://www.cdc.gov/ncbddd/hemophilia/data.html>.

their own supply of clotting factor to Camp. It comes in glass flasks packed in cardboard boxes that are quite bulky, and it requires refrigeration. After only a few summers when the boxes of clotting Factor exceeded the Infirmary refrigeration capacity, we purchased a large commercial refrigerator to accommodate this particular need.

Before 1985, the Factor VIII concentrates used for treatment of Hemophilia A were prepared by combining plasma from as many as 25,000 individual donors, and they often were contaminated with the Human Immunodeficiency Virus (HIV). Many boys with hemophilia died of Acquired Immunodeficiency Syndrome (AIDS) after receiving contaminated Factor VIII concentrates. This is no longer a threat because Factor VIII concentrates are now manufactured using recombinant DNA technology, which eliminates the risk of contamination by any type of virus. Today, Factor IX concentrates are also produced using recombinant DNA technology.

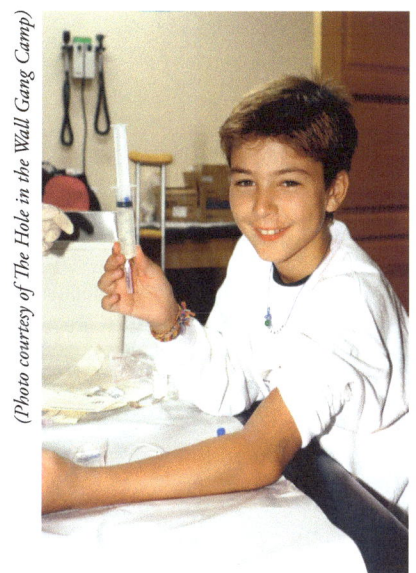

Self-administration of Factor concentrate

(Photo courtesy of The Hole in the Wall Gang Camp)

An important advance has been the recent discovery that Factor VIII or Factor IX concentrates can be administered three to four times a week prophylactically, even if there is no clinical bleeding. When this is done, the level of the Factor is sufficient to prevent most clinical bleeding episodes. Today, about three-quarters of the campers with hemophilia are receiving this prophylactic therapy despite its great expense. Some of these boys have permanent "internal ports" to facilitate Factor administration; and many learn to self-administer, enhancing their independence.

A typical Camp session usually includes 15 to 20 boys with hemophilia. In the community, a boy with hemophilia experiencing a bleeding episode usually goes to an Emergency Room or is hospitalized for treatment. At THITWGC, hemophilic bleeding episodes can be treated on site by injection of the appropriate Factor concentrates. This has permitted boys with hemophilia and campers with other conditions requiring treatment to fully participate in Camp activities, including horseback riding, climbing the Tower, descending on the zip line, and participating in the Challenge Course.

Sickle cell anemia is predominantly a disease of African-Americans, although some children of Italian or Greek ancestry and some from western hemisphere Hispanic families also have this genetic disease. An individual with only one sickle cell gene has asymptomatic sickle cell trait. When both parents have sickle cell trait and each gives their baby a sickle cell gene, the baby develops the full disease of sickle cell anemia. About two million people in the U.S. have sickle cell trait. There are somewhere between 70,000 and 100,000 people in the United States with sickle cell anemia, and an estimated one in 500 African-American newborns has the disease.[5] Red blood cells are normally round, soft, and flexible little donuts. But with sickle cell anemia, the red blood cells may become elongated and rigid. Because of this shape, they have difficulty passing through small blood vessels and can block blood flow, creating a logjam. When this happens, the part of

---

5   National Heart, Lung, and Blood Institute, 2014 <http://www.nhlbi.nih.gov/health/health-topics/topics/sca/atrisk>.

the body tissue beyond the blockade is deprived of oxygen and may be damaged. This can result in severe pain in the body tissue that is not receiving oxygen, and it can occur in any part of the body. When this happens, it is called a "pain crisis." There is no specific treatment for the sickle cell pain crisis beyond managing the symptoms and assuring adequate hydration. Pain medications, ranging from acetaminophen and ibuprofen to codeine and morphine, may be needed. Another type of sickle cell anemia is hemoglobin SC disease, which is usually less severe clinically.

When I was treating sickle cell anemia patients in the 1960's, the mean life expectancy was only about 15 years, and survival above 50 years of age was unusual. A major contributor to the short life span was the fact that about 25% of infants born with sickle cell anemia died in their first five years of life.[6] Most of these children died of sudden, overwhelming bacterial infections. At the time, neonatal screening was available to identify newborns with sickle cell anemia, but it was used only to determine the frequency of the disease. There was usually no comprehensive follow-up provided. In many cases, death was the first recognized clinical manifestation of sickle cell anemia in a young child.

I reasoned that although I could not cure sickle cell anemia, I could successfully treat young children and prevent their untimely deaths by early identification and new management protocols. This led to my establishing a program for neonatal diagnosis in New Haven in 1972. Since virtually all children in the United States are born in a hospital, neonatal diagnosis can be readily accomplished. In 1972-1973, 756 African-American newborns at Yale-New Haven Hospital were screened. Six of them (0.8%) had sickle cell anemia.[7]

To assess the effect of neonatal screening accompanied by an aggressive follow-up effort, a Yale medical student and I reviewed State of Connecticut death certificates in two periods: 1) Between 1970 and 1988, when there was no state-wide neonatal screening, and 2) Between 1990 and 2002, when there was universal neonatal testing by the State Department of Health laboratory. In the first period, there were 13 deaths, most of which were associated with infections. In the second period, there were no deaths.[8] We had successfully demonstrated that neonatal diagnosis, combined with prophylactic antibiotics, immunizations, careful follow-up, and hospital admission if a child developed a fever, essentially eliminated early deaths from infection. Because of our work, the standard of practice became close follow-up of newborns identified with sickle cell anemia. The average life expectancy for people with sickle cell anemia is now about 45 years, with survival above 50 years of age becoming more common.[9] Neonatal screening for sickle cell anemia is now performed by almost all state health departments in the United States during the neonatal period because of the proven benefits of early diagnosis.

During the first year of THITWGC, children with sickle cell anemia attended the general sessions. Although our general sessions still have campers with this disease, during the third year

---

6 L Diggs, et al., "Anatomic Lesions in Sickle Cell Diseases," *In Sickle Cell Diseases*, Editors H. Abramson, et al., (St. Louis: C.V. Mosby Co., 1973) 218-219.

7 HA Pearson, et al., "Routine screening of umbilical cord blood for sickle cell diseases," *Journal of the American Medical Association* 227 (1974): 420-421.

8 T Frempong and HA Pearson, "Newborn screening coupled with comprehensive follow up reduced early mortality of sickle cell disease in Connecticut," *Connecticut Medicine* 71 (2007): 9-12.

9 O Platt, et al., "Mortality in sickle cell disease—Life expectancy and risk factors for early death," *New England Journal of Medicine* 330 (1994): 1639-1644.

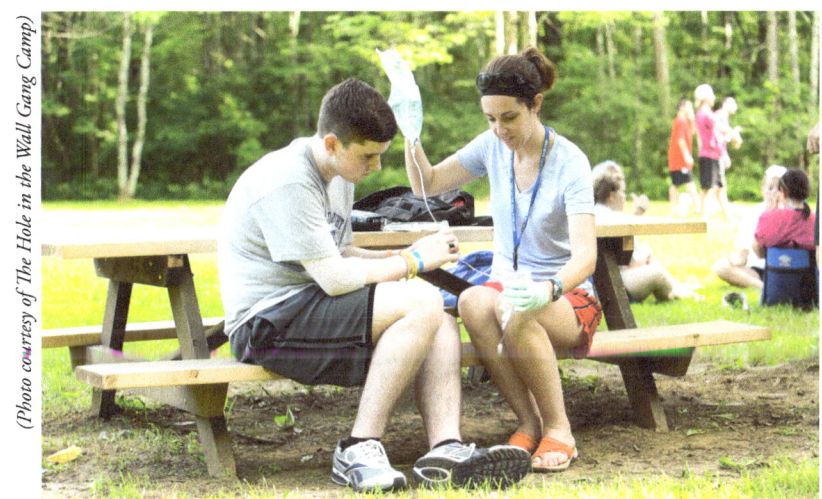
(Photo courtesy of The Hole in the Wall Gang Camp)

Receiving medication at an outdoor activity

(1990) we instituted Sickle Cell Special Sessions, which are explained below. Because more children with sickle cell anemia now survive past early childhood, there are consistently high numbers of campers with this condition each year.

Thalassemia major research during the past several decades has increased the life expectancy of individuals with this disease, and premarital testing for thalassemia trait and genetic counseling have reduced its prevalence. Dotty Guiliotis and I were active in these aspects of thalassemia in the New Haven area. This disease, also called "Cooley's Anemia," primarily occurs in Mediterranean populations (Italian, Greek, and middle-Eastern) but also extends into some Asian areas of the world. The word "thalassemia" is derived from the Latin words for "sea in the blood" and refers to the fact that it centers in the regions surrounding the Mediterranean Sea. The disease was given the eponym for Thomas B. Cooley, a pediatric hematologist in Detroit, who first described the disease in 1925.[10] In 2014, there were an estimated 1,000 people in the United States with thalassemia major.[11] The initial symptom is anemia appearing in the first three or four months of life. The anemia becomes so severe that death is likely unless regular monthly blood transfusions are given. The child usually does well with the transfusions for several years. However, over time, the iron from the transfused blood builds up and causes organ damage, particularly in the heart.

In the past, children with thalassemia died in their teens or early twenties due to iron overload. In the 1970s, hematologists began using desferoxamine, an injected medication that picks up (chelates) the iron from the blood so that it can be excreted in the urine. To be effective, the medication had to be slowly injected under the skin over an extended period of time, usually during sleep at least five nights a week, using a special battery-driven pump designed by Dean Kamen, the brother of one of Yale's pediatric residents. This treatment extended life expectancy of people with thalassemia into their thirties and forties, but there was often poor patient compliance with this rigorous regimen. More recently, an oral iron-chelating agent (deferipron) has been developed. It was used extensively in European patients with thalassemia major and shown to be

---

10 Wikipedia, 2014 <http.//en.wikipedia.org/wiki/Thomas_Benton_Cooley>
11 Wikipedia, 2014 <http://en.wikipedia.org/wiki/Thalassemia>

effective. However, because of concerns about possible toxicities, it was not approved for use in the United States until 2011. Its use, in conjunction with other oral chelators, facilitates increased patient adherence to therapy and better health.

Developing effective therapies is only part of the challenge. The other part is reaching out to the populations affected by the disease. Dotty Guiliotis and I worked together to streamline and improve the care for children with thalassemia and their families in the New Haven area. I frequently went to the Greek churches or Dotty's home to draw the blood of children to save families either extra trips to the hospital or long waits for the blood typing and cross matching prior to blood transfusions. From 1972 to 1974, Dotty and I conducted a comprehensive screening and counseling program for thalassemia trait. Working through the three large Greek Orthodox parishes in Connecticut, we drew blood and tested for the trait on more than 600 people. We identified 75 individuals with thalassemia trait and provided them with education and genetic counseling. We also tested family members of these individuals with thalassemia trait and found an additional 17 people with the trait. With this knowledge, many people with the trait made marriage and family planning choices to avoid having children with thalassemia major. As a result, about 40 years later, there are no longer cases of thalassemia major being diagnosed in our local Greek community. We believe that screening at-risk populations and providing early, effective genetic counseling can reduce the frequency of new cases of thalassemia major.[12] Several years ago, Dotty was told by a priest visiting from Greece that because they had learned of our research, the Orthodox priests in Greece were facilitating premarital screening for thalassemia trait followed by counseling for couples when both had the trait. When camper recruitment began in 1988, I included my patients with thalassemia major, and a good number of them benefitted from Camp. Some of them later became counselors.

There are occasionally children with rare inherited anemias at THITWGC. Congenital hypoplastic anemia (Diamond Blackfan Syndrome) falls into this category. Before the mid-1950s, it was treated with regular blood transfusions.[13] This disease sparked my interest in becoming a pediatric hematologist back in 1957, when I reported the first American case that responded to corticosteroid therapy and no longer required transfusions. At that time, I was a pediatric resident at the U. S. Naval Hospital in Bethesda, Maryland. I later became a pediatric hematology fellow at Boston Children's Hospital under the guidance of Dr. Louis Diamond, for whom the disease is named. Another disease in this category is hereditary spherocytosis, an autosomal dominant genetic blood disease, which means that one of the parents has the condition. It often appears in the newborn period with hyperbilirubinemia (too much bilirubin resulting in jaundice, or yellowing of the skin and eyes) and causes severe anemia because the spherocytic red blood cells are trapped and destroyed, primarily in the spleen. A splenectomy (removing the spleen), usually after four years of age, can cure hereditary spherocytosis. Because there is a cure, children with this condition are only occasionally campers. Another category of rare inherited anemias is called congenital non-spherocytic (hemolytic) anemia. There are several enzymatic defects that cause this disorder, including glucose-6-phophate dehydrogenase (G6PD) and pyruvate kinase deficiencies.

---

12   HA Pearson, et al., "Thalassemia in Greek Americans", *Journal of Pediatrics* 86 (1975), pp 917-918.

13   HA Pearson and TE Cone, "Congenital hypoplastic anemia," *Pediatrics* 19 (1957): 192-200.

Although these are chronic diseases that do not respond to splenectomy, the anemia is usually not severe.

There are periodically children at Camp with other blood diseases that are autoimmune, meaning that an individual develops antibodies which attack the body's own cells. The most common autoimmune blood disease in children is idiopathic thrombocytopenic purpura (ITP), which is caused by an auto antibody that destroys the blood platelets. As a result, children with ITP have a low platelet count that results in easy bruising and bleeding. It usually runs a course of several weeks or months and can be controlled by corticosteroid medication. In about 25% of cases, it becomes a chronic disease that may be treated by splenectomy and immunotherapy.

Another autoimmune blood disease in children is aplastic anemia, a disease in which the bone marrow loses its capacity to manufacture the essential elements of the blood—red blood cells, white blood cells, and platelets. In some cases, aplastic anemia is caused by an auto antibody that attacks the bone marrow stem cells. It might also be the result of toxic damage to the bone marrow, perhaps from medication (particularly chloramphenicol, no longer used in the United States), radiation, or other environmental exposures; but many times a cause is not identified. Its usual treatment for many years was bone marrow transplantation, a complicated and risky procedure. We used to have campers each year who received bone marrow transplants for this disease as well as for a variety of other diseases. Now, children with aplastic anemia are more likely to receive anti-thymocyte globulin (ATG) and immuno-suppression therapies.

Autoimmune hemolytic anemia (AHA) and autoimmune neutropenia are two rare immunologic blood diseases. In AHA, the patient's body develops antibodies that cause destruction of red blood cells. If there is immunologic destruction of white blood cells (neutrophils), neutropenia is the diagnosis. Children with AHA develop anemia, and those with autoimmune neutropenia are susceptible to bacterial infections. These diseases are usually self-limited. If they become chronic, corticosteroids, immunotherapy, and splenectomy are therapies for both conditions.

Other Diseases

Each year we accept a number of children who do not meet the diagnostic criteria of cancer and blood diseases. We will accept children with other diseases if they are not able to attend a regular summer camp. Some of these diseases are described below.

- Human Immune-deficiency Virus (HIV) and Acquired Immune-Deficiency Syndrome (AIDS): HIV/AIDS is an infectious disease caused by a virus affecting the body's immune system that can result in severe, life-threatening infections and early death. A newborn can acquire the virus from an HIV-positive mother. Contaminated blood or blood products can also transmit the disease, as it did in the past to boys with hemophilia. HIV at Camp is addressed more extensively in the Special Sessions section.
- Congenital immunodeficiencies, inherited abnormalities in the immune system: Children born with these disorders have increased risk of infection throughout life. They are often treated with a medication called Intravenous Immunoglobulin (IVIG), which is given over several hours.

- Metabolic disorders (inborn errors of metabolism), inherited conditions that affect how the human body breaks down food and converts it to energy: In these disorders, specific substances that the body needs might be too low, too high, or missing completely, causing serious medical problems. These diseases are often treated prophylactically with regular infusions with the missing substance. In recent years, Medical Director Dr. Sharon Space has been instrumental in bringing children with these disorders to Camp.
- Orphan diseases so rare that fewer than five in every 10,000 people have them: Orphan diseases can cause serious health issues and require complicated medical treatment. Camp accepts children with orphan diseases for general sessions but also reaches out to families during Family Weekends. At a 2014 Camp Family Weekend, there were two families with children with Progeria, an extremely rare disease associated with early and accelerated aging. Progeria is a fatal disease with an average life span of 13 years. There are only about 200 to 250 children with Progeria alive in the world at any one time.[14] In early 2015, there were about 18 living in the United States.[15] In the summer of 2015, Camp hosted a Progeria Family Weekend, the first of its kind in the United States, with 11 of the 20 known families from the U.S. and Canada participating. The ages of the children ranged from three to 14 years. Dr. Space reflected,

> "It was an incredible weekend! It reminded me of the early days when we first started serving kids with HIV. The children, their parents, and their siblings were finally part of a community where they did not look different than everybody else. They were in a place where they were completely accepted, valued, and celebrated and where everyone understood what they were going through. The 'stares' the kids got were not because they looked different but because the kids had never seen so many people who look the same as they do. It was a very powerful experience."

In the summer of 2001, we had a camper with a benign lymphatic tumor of her neck, another example of a diagnosis that does not meet the standard criteria of cancer or a life-threatening blood disease. While the tumor did not metastasize, the bulk of it had to be surgically removed, only to grow back and once again cause problems in breathing and eating. The child had a tracheostomy to allow her to breathe. The girl's nurse had submitted an application along with a request to personally bring her patient to Camp from New Jersey and participate as a nursing volunteer for the session. When she came to Camp, the child was allowed to swim in a pool for the very first time. Both the camper and her nurse had an unforgettable experience.

No matter what the diagnoses are in a given session, with the volume of campers it is essential to have medical protocols and systems in place along with adequate numbers of trained medical and nursing professionals. Prior to the start of the session, the medical and nursing staff members review the medical files and assign campers to a cabin in one of the five Units. As children and their families converge upon Camp at each session's beginning, the resident clowns, counselors, nurses, and other staff are ready and waiting for them. There are about 120 to 130 children and their families to greet for each session, and many of the campers require medications and special

---

14 Progeria Research Foundation, 2014 <http://progeriaresearch.org/progeria_101.html>.
15 Unpublished data, Brianna J O'Connell, MS, CCLS, Boston Children's Hospital, Boston, MA.

accommodations because of their illnesses. After entering Camp, families are directed to park near the Horse Barn, get their Unit assignment, and check in with their Unit nurse. Unit nurses each have a caseload of about 25 to 30 campers. At check-in, they review the medical status with the family and often learn of additional needs or concerns about the child at that time. The nurses collect and label medications, utilizing a basket system for safe sorting and keeping. When families have to wait for the Unit nurse, clowns and other staff keep them engaged and entertained.

After check-in, the campers are transported by golf cart or walk to their cabin to meet their counselors and cabin mates. Parents are directed to the Dining Hall for food. For first-time families, veteran parents are available for questions and emotional support. A Dining Hall gathering for parents occurs at the conclusion of the session as well, when parents might have to cope with children who do not want to leave Camp!

By the end of the first day of a session, medical and nursing routines kick into place. During the day, Unit nurses dispense medications at meals in the Dining Hall. For the few campers needing additional bedtime doses, nurses provide them in the Infirmary or in the cabins. When a medical concern or question arises at night, a cabin counselor will phone the nurse or physician on night call, as assigned by the Medical and Nursing Directors. Medical and nursing staff and volunteers are accommodated in housing near the Infirmary. Additional volunteer nurses are assigned to Units with particularly demanding medical needs to provide extra help. Unit nurses are given cell phones to use in case of special arising needs or emergencies. During the day, they accompany their campers to activities. Their presence allows them to keep on top of their campers' health and medical needs. There is always at least one nurse and one physician in or nearby the Infirmary. The ready availability of the golf cart fleet assures a quick response in case of an emergency.

Camp has been fortunate to have competent, experienced, dedicated nursing leadership over the years. When Sue Johnson left in 1999, she was succeeded by Karen Molloy, who had volunteered in 1995 and then served as Staff Nurse for four summers. Karen held the Nursing Director position for eight years, from 2000 to 2007. Patti Carlton served as Nursing Director from 2007 to 2011, and Juli Mason has been in the position from 2012 to the present (2015).

With a skillfully designed Camp, highly competent staff and volunteers, efficient systems for responding to medical needs of both campers and staff, and extraordinary levels of enthusiasm and energy, Camp is truly a place where our children can be safe while "raising a little hell" as Paul wanted.

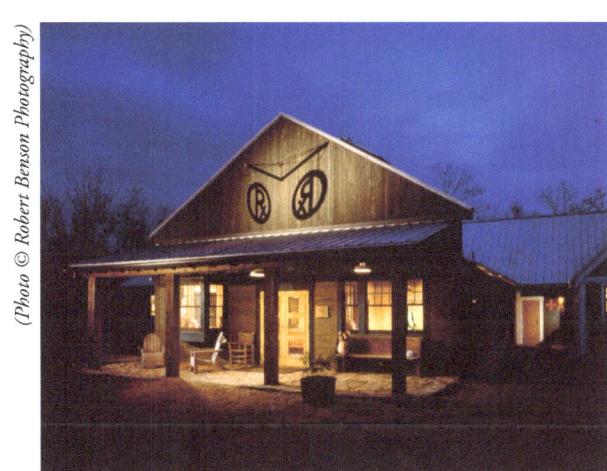

The OK Corral Infirmary at night

CHAPTER NINE

Special Sessions

Immunology Sessions

> *"I originally intended Camp to be for kids with cancer but even before it opened, we expanded that mission to include serious blood disorders and other life-threatening diseases. I think we were the first residential camp that publicly took HIV positive kids. In the mid-1980s, there wasn't much knowledge about HIV/AIDS. I think the community could have been nervous about having kids with AIDS at Camp, but Doc Pearson reassured the town fathers that there was no risk. There were no objections from the medical community. As with all the campers, it wasn't the doctors we had to convince, it was the mothers and fathers."* – Paul Newman

In 1988, the very first year, a camper with hemophilia came to Camp. His application did not mention that he had HIV/AIDS and had suffered from several opportunistic infections. His HIV was being treated in an experimental program at the National Institutes of Health (NIH) and not at his usual clinic in Florida. Sue became aware of this when she talked to his family when they delivered him to THITWGC on June 18. I was concerned that we had not told the staff or families that there could be campers with AIDS at Camp. This was a time when there was a lot of misinformation, concern, and even hysteria about AIDS. I decided not to send the camper home and had him assigned to a cabin in one of the Units. I assembled the whole staff and very calmly explained that there was none to minimal danger to them personally if simple precautions were exercised. I carefully outlined those precautions. I offered to reassign the counselors of the cabin where the boy was to be placed, but none of them asked for this.

I then called the parents of the other campers assigned to the cabin where the boy would be staying and explained the situation to them. Two questions were asked:

1. "How had the boy developed AIDS?" I explained that he had hemophilia and had been infected by injections of virus-contaminated clotting factor prescribed by his doctors to treat bleeding episodes.
2. "What is the risk to my child if he interacts with the boy and sleeps in the same room?" I told them that AIDS can only be transmitted by exposure to blood and that there would be ample supervision and care to prevent this from happening.

I offered to have their child moved to another cabin, but all of them declined. During the rest of the summer and the next summer, a number of other boys with hemophilia who were HIV-positive came to Camp. There were no repercussions.

Children who had been infected with the HIV virus at birth from infected mothers (vertical transmission) were being diagnosed in substantial numbers in the late 1980s and were being followed in clinics in large urban areas. HIV/AIDS was of very great public concern at the time. Children were being barred from school and families isolated because of HIV. I felt that these children, many of whom were orphans because their parents had died, were in great need of the kind of experience that Camp could provide and explored the possibility of having a special session for children with vertically transmitted HIV/AIDS.

I did not go into a special HIV/AIDS session blindly because I knew that it was a fairly daring venture that required a lot of advance planning. I did research and consulted infectious disease experts. They unanimously reassured me that there was not a significant risk of casual exposure if we all exercised careful observation and followed rather minimal precautions, as I had told the staff in June, 1988. I contacted some of the centers in New York where these children were being followed and was told that they were excited about the possibility of a special session at Camp that their patients might attend. They also said that their staff members might accompany the children en route and help with their care at Camp.

I cleared the plan with the District and State Boards of Health, and nobody had objections. Because many of the children were orphans and wards of other states, we made special arrangements to get permission to bring them to Camp, to have them cross state lines, and to treat them if necessary. Transportation by buses had to be provided to bring the children to Camp and return them home at the end of the session.

Some of the parents and their physicians expressed concern that a child might be stigmatized by going to an HIV/AIDS session, so cameras and photographs were not allowed and children were not identified by name. Finally, it was not called an "HIV/AIDS Session" but rather an "Immunology Session,"[1] something of a euphemism!

I realized that it was essential to inform the neighboring townspeople that many children infected with HIV/AIDS would be coming to THITWGC. If we tried to do this surreptitiously, it surely would leak out and we might have neighbors marching into Camp with torches! I invited leaders of Ashford and Eastford to a luncheon at Camp, ostensibly to bring them generally up to date. I made a list of things to cover at the meeting; for example, Camp has been a very good

---

1 HA Pearson, et al., "Residential summer camp for children with vertically transmitted HIV/AIDS—A six-year experience at the Hole in the Wall Gang Camp," *Pediatrics* 100 (1997): 709-713.

neighbor, we preferentially hire workers and vendors from the immediate area, we make yearly contributions to our towns in lieu of property taxes, etc., etc. I presented this list; but in the middle, I mentioned that we were going to have children with HIV at Camp and that there were no risks to them. No objections or comments were made.

The first Immunology Session, which we considered to be a pilot session, was held in mid-August 1989. Forty HIV-positive children, aged six to 12 years, were transported to Camp from their home medical centers in Connecticut, New York and New Jersey. The average camper was receiving two or three oral medications, and five nurses were present to facilitate dispensing them. The pilot session went well, without incidents and to the great joy of the children. It was decided to make Immunology Sessions a regular part of the summer schedule. This was the first residential camp for HIV positive children in New England and one of the first in the world, something that makes me very proud.

Children diagnosed with HIV/AIDS often lose their appetites to the point of becoming emaciated. Camp consistently provides a varied menu with foods and beverages that children like, including cold cereals, pizza, hamburgers, pasta, chocolate milk, and lemonade (but no sodas). This same fare is offered during the Immunology Sessions, and most of the children eat with enthusiasm. In 1991, pediatrician Dr. Antonia Novello, the United States Surgeon General during Bill Clinton's presidency, visited Camp for two days during the Immunology Session. Dr. Novello had extensive experience with children with HIV, having served as Chair of the Department of Health and Human Services Task Force for Children and HIV in the United States. Pleasantly surprised at the appetites, Dr. Novello exclaimed, "People won't believe that these children have HIV if you look at the way they eat!" At Camp, we attribute healthy appetites to be a result of both the tasty food, the singing and dancing after meals in the Dining Hall, and the entire Camp experience of the fun activities in which children participate.

In the 1995 Immunology Session, there were 100 campers who represented an estimated 20% of the six- to 15-year-old children with vertically transmitted HIV in the entire USA! Despite this, many children who wanted to attend could not be accommodated. In an attempt to address this, two Immunology Sessions were held in the summers from 1996 to 2009. Between 1993 and 1996, the number of medications that needed to be dispensed escalated to include retroviral, protease inhibitors, prophylactic antibacterial, anti-fungal and anti-pneumocystis agents, and many others. In the two 1996 Immunology Sessions, *the number of medication types per camper* ranged from none to 22, with an average of 4.5. *Total daily administrations per child* ranged from none to 27, with an average of 7.5. As the number of medications the campers required escalated, there was a concomitant increase in nursing workload that required an increase of nurses. Beginning in 1993, the number of nurses was increased from five to ten, including seven volunteer nurses. Two additional physicians with HIV/AIDS experience and one or two senior pediatric residents made up the medical staff. Some of the children had special medical problems that we addressed in ways to best accommodate them as campers. Overnight intravenous nutrition (hyper alimentation) was given in the cabins. One child had overnight peritoneal dialysis in his cabin. Oxygen therapy equipment was available, including a digital pulse oximeter and a nebulizer for inhalation therapy.

The Immunology Sessions should soon be phased out. Boys with hemophilia have had access to safe Factor infusions for many years, virtually eliminating new HIV/AIDS diagnoses among them. The number of children being born with HIV is decreasing sharply because of the increased detection and perinatal treatment of HIV-infected mothers. By 2010, there were so few children of camping age with vertically transmitted HIV that there was only one Immunology Session. Soon none will be needed. With advances in HIV/AIDS treatments, many former campers are thriving more than two decades after being infected. What great progress!

Sickle Cell Sessions

> *"A marvelous African American girl with sickle cell anemia told me that coming to Camp was what she lived for. She said that why she stayed alive for 11 ½ months was to be able to come to Camp in the summer."* – Paul Newman

Children with sickle cell anemia were accepted as campers from the very first summer because of the seriousness of this blood disease. Initially, most of these children came from centers in Connecticut and Rhode Island. I knew that there were thousands of children with sickle cell disease in metropolitan Boston, New York, New Jersey, and Pennsylvania. I realized that if we tried to take too many of them as campers, we could become a sickle cell camp. However, because there were so many of them in our catchment area, I wanted to serve more of them at THITWGC without straying too much of our original mission focusing on children with cancer. I decided to start with a special Sickle Cell Session for children from Metropolitan New York City and Northern New Jersey. During the spring of 1990, I visited sickle cell centers in these cities and talked with clinic directors, most of whom I knew. We planned to bring 100 children recruited by the centers to Camp for a seven-day session in mid-July. THITWGC arranged for buses to transport the children as well as a number of clinic staff who came as volunteers from their clinics to Camp.

The first Sickle Cell Session was held in July 1990 and was attended by 90 campers, providing a residential camping experience for urban children who did not have a lot of other opportunities. Despite having studied and treated patients with sickle cell anemia for several decades, I gained new perspectives by living with a hundred children with sickle cell anemia 24 hours a day for a week. The pain crises that these children have can be devastating and more frequent than I thought from my hospital experience.

I have taught over the years that most of the time we do not know what precipitates a pain crisis, but at Camp I definitely learned that swimming in cool water can be the cause. During the first Sickle Cell Session, many campers were brought to the infirmary directly from the Swimming Pool complaining of such severe pain in their arms and legs that narcotic treatment was often necessary. When we checked the pool water temperature, we found that it was at times below 70º F, too cold for our children. We decided to heat the pool water between 85º and 90º. Because I observed that children often shivered when they came out of the heated pool, I had George Harakaly build a poolside gazebo enclosed by Plexiglas and with infrared heat lamps in the ceiling. The counselors named it the "French Fryer." When the children and counselors leave the pool, they go into the French Fryer, where they stay warm while drying off. During the Sickle Cell

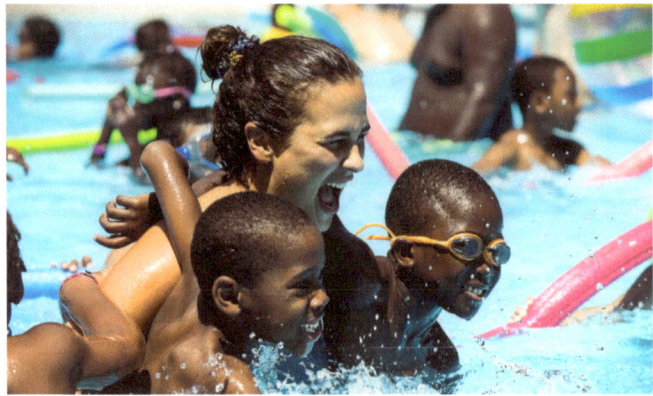
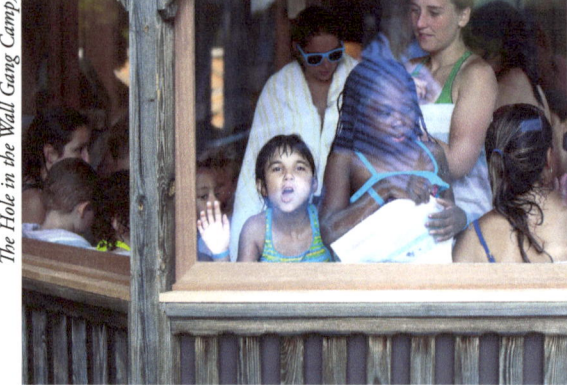

Enjoying the Swimming Pool *Warming up in the French Fryer*

(Both photos courtesy of The Hole in the Wall Gang Camp)

Sessions, there are wall-to-wall children in the pool enjoying swimming, often for the first time. After increasing the water temperature of the pool and installing the French Fryer, pain episodes associated with swimming virtually disappeared.

The Sickle Cell Sessions were so successful that in 2002 they were increased to two sessions and included children from Boston and Philadelphia. During most summers, Camp serves over 300 children with a diagnosis of sickle cell anemia.

Brother and Sister (Sibling) Sessions

Having worked with children with cancer and life threatening diseases and their families for a long time, I knew well from personal experience that the healthy brothers and sisters of kids with these serious diseases often, and understandably, may be pushed aside. The parents are so invested and involved with the ill child and his/her treatments that the healthy children in the family can be marginalized. Being unintentionally ignored by the people who should love you the most can be confusing. I decided that THITWGC should try to do something special for these children, who often get overlooked and can develop behavioral problems or begin failing in school.

There were three possibilities. We could have a family camping session, but our facilities at the time were not designed for families. We could have a session where both regular campers and their healthy siblings would be at Camp together. Finally, we could have a special session for only the healthy brothers and sisters. I posed these options to the parents of some of our regular campers, and almost unanimously they responded, "Let the siblings go to Camp by themselves so they can be the center of attention and be special." In 1991, we had our first Brother and Sister Session, and these have continued. I did not want to call it the "Sibling Session" because it sounded too clinical!

To me, it has been successful because when the healthy siblings return home from Camp, they bring a common though not shared experience with the ill children. They talk to each other about Camp saying, "I went fishing and caught a big bass," with the other responding, "So did I!" The Brother and Sister Sessions are one of the most innovative things that I have done at Camp. It was the first THITWGC program serving the extended Camp family. Other such programs subsequently developed are the COPE program for parents mentioned later and the spring and fall

Family Weekends.

One family in particular comes to my mind when I reflect on how THITWGC changed their lives and, in turn, how they have given back to Camp. This story is told with their permission. When Danny was diagnosed with cancer, his sister Ana was ten years old. Danny's illness and their parents' attempts to protect Ana began a period of emotional challenges for her that involved confusion, loneliness, and increasing anger. Ana began rebelling in school. A couple of years after his diagnosis and treatment, Danny attended Camp for the first time. Ana accompanied her father to pick Danny up at the end of the session, and she felt a turn of emotions as they drove through the gate and she saw what she referred to as "Crazy People" waving brightly colored streamers, blowing giant bubbles, and jumping to wild music. They made her laugh. As she related in an interview with Timothy Hotchner:

> "One of these Crazy People asked me if I wanted a name tag and I said, 'Yes, my name is Danny's sister.' My first impulse was to be a smart aleck, but these people, instead of looking at me with pity and saying, 'You're more than that,' this Crazy Person saw the truth in that statement and replied with, 'What an interesting name! How do you spell that?'"

Ana distinctly felt that Camp was special and had a very positive effect on her brother. She also felt her anger return. At the end of that summer, she attended the Brother & Sister Session. At one point she felt so confused by her emotions that she asked one of the counselors to take a walk with her. On the walk to the Memory Garden, Ana cried, and the counselor held her. Ana later related:

> "I hadn't been held in so long that I got so overwhelmed and burst into tears. Jenny let me cry and for someone who took it upon herself to be strong all the time, this was huge. In those moments I grew up, not in the way a precocious teenager wants to, but the way that a healthy adult has to. The Hole in the Wall Gang Camp gave me reason to stop being angry…Not only was I thankful for Danny, but I was thankful for everything that happened thereafter…Even if the illness doesn't inhabit our bodies, it infects our minds in ways that medicine cannot heal…Recently, I sat in on multiple interviews about ways in which Camp has affected and saved so many families. I found myself particularly attuned to the sibling stories. While most of the interviews focused on the illness-affected child, one mother made a brief comment on how she was worried about her sibling son…When the mother added that her son would be going to Sibling Camp for the first time, I immediately felt relieved…I can say that Camp brought about a monumental change and a new perspective that will forever be at the forefront of my never-ending journey toward emotional recovery."

Danny and Ana's father, Dr. Richard Kayne, is a physician, Board member, and COPE volunteer (explained later). His oldest child, Michael, has been a Camp volunteer. Richard has given much of his time and energy back to Camp, but like many of us, he will say that he has received much more than he has given. Richard is known at Camp for his eagerness to talk with and listen to families and for his crazy hats. His presence emits positive energy, and his hats give us joy.

Because I spent so much of my time at Camp during the summers between 1988 and 2002, THITWGC became an important part in the lives of three generations of my own family. In many cases, their involvement began during the Brother and Sister Session. Oftentimes, the only way Anne and I saw grandchildren during the summer was at Camp. Although cabin priority was given to siblings of campers, when beds were available, my grandchildren were allowed to participate. Andrew, Alex, Katy, Sarah, Annemarie, Palomita, Johnny, Siobhan, Sile, Damon, and Seana came to Camp during sibling sessions. While they all enjoyed the fun times, my grandchildren also developed the understanding of Camp's purpose and empathy for the families involved. That was true as well for grandsons Matthew and Daniel, who participated during general sessions while their parents Stephen and Mary Lou were volunteers.

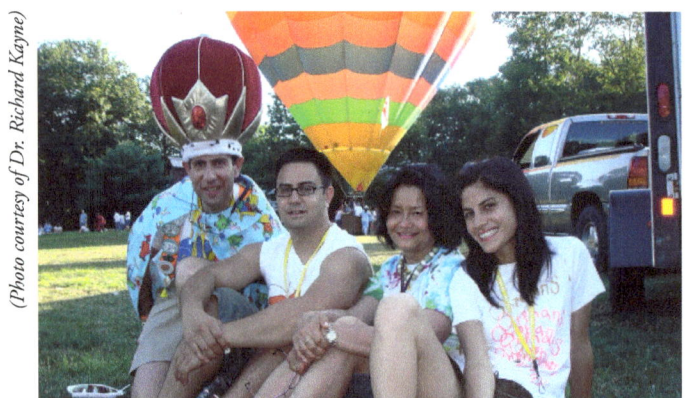

The Kayne Family: Richard (in crazy hat), Danny, Maria (mother), and Ana (Michael is not present)

(Photo courtesy of Dr. Richard Kayne)

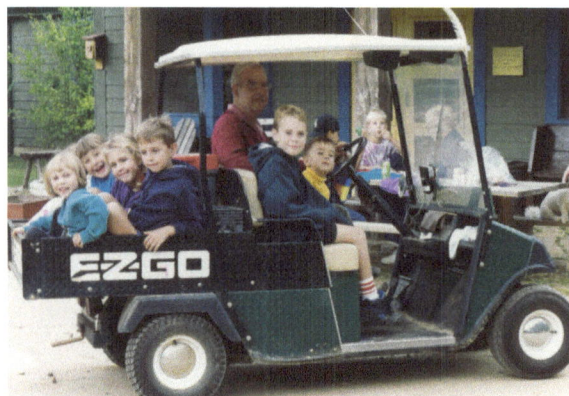

With some of my grandchildren at their first visit to Camp in 1992

CHAPTER TEN

Reflecting on Camp's Past and Looking to the Future

In addition to the regular summer camping experience, THITWGC has grown to offer a variety of outreach programs to children and their families. These additional programs, all offered at no cost to participants, maximize the utilization of the Camp facilities and staff for the benefit of the children and families. Reunion Weekends provide a chance for children to maintain their friendships during the fall when Camp is not in session. Family Weekends provide a special opportunity for ill children and their entire families to experience the magic of THITWGC. They occur during some of the spring and fall weekends when Camp is not in session.

COPE (Change of Pace Experience) is a program held over a weekend at a hotel for parents of first-time summer campers. Several sessions of COPE are offered each year, providing respite, renewal, laughter, and fun, as well as an opportunity for sharing experiences and developing friendships with parents of other campers. Originally, it was a group discussion program for parents of children with cancer set up by Barbara Johanson, a social worker in Greenwich Hospital in Connecticut. In 1990, Barbara transferred her program to Camp, where it was organized by Knettie Archard and Karen Allen, original Camp staff members. COPE allows the parents of campers to spend time together and then return to their children refreshed, strengthened and, most importantly, no longer feeling alone. Dr. Richard Kayne has participated in and helped facilitate COPE for a number of years. In 2014, there were five COPE sessions with 40 to 70 attendees each.

My good friend and long-time Camp volunteer Father Domenic (Dom) Roscioli, himself a cancer survivor, has been with COPE from its beginning. Many years ago, when Father Dom was initially diagnosed with cancer, his Bishop allowed him to go home with the belief that he did not have much time left on this Earth. Back at home in Wisconsin, he began doing community work. Among his projects was the establishment of a company that produced and sold "Father Dom's Duck's Doo Compost—Food for the Soil," fertilizer made from duck poop. (Others have referred to it as "Soul for the Soil.") The profits go to charity. Father Dom first learned about Camp in 1988 through an article in the Chicago press. He called Camp and was invited to volunteer, which he has been doing since 1989.

The Hospital Outreach Program (HOP) takes Camp's creative activities, including art and woodworking, into over 30 hospitals in New England, New York, New Jersey, and Pennsylvania to improve the quality of life for children undergoing treatment of their life-threatening diseases. Launched in 2014, the Camp Out Program uses a specially equipped, colorful van to take Arts & Crafts to New England children who are homebound due to their illnesses. With all of its programs taken into account, Camp is currently serving about 30,000 people each year.

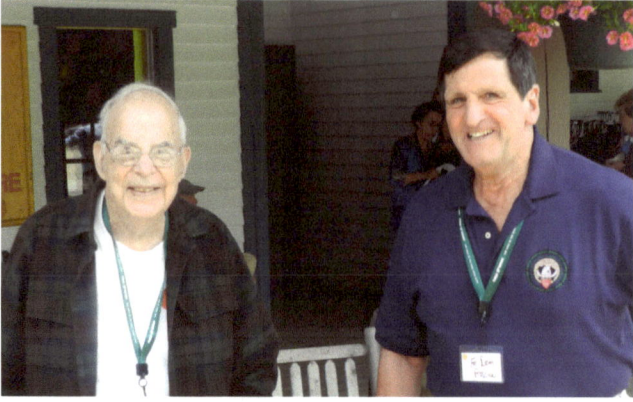

With Father Dom in 2013

Program activities have continued to evolve. Camp now has a tennis court, miniature golf, archery range, and a baseball field. A climbing wall has been installed in the Gymnasium. During the second from the last day of each Brother and Sister Session, a camp-wide "capture the flag" game is played. Campers are divided into two groups, each of which is given a flag to defend. They have a rowdy time trying to capture the flag of the other group. I have faith in the creativity of staff and campers to continue introducing new programs and traditions in the future.

Fundraising continues each year to support THITWGC and its array of on-site and off-site programs. About half of Camp's budget comes from individual donations and proceeds from the Galas, with the other half coming from businesses and foundations. More information on THITWGC can be found at www.holeinthewallgang.org and on the Newman's Own Foundation website at www.newmansownfoundation.org.

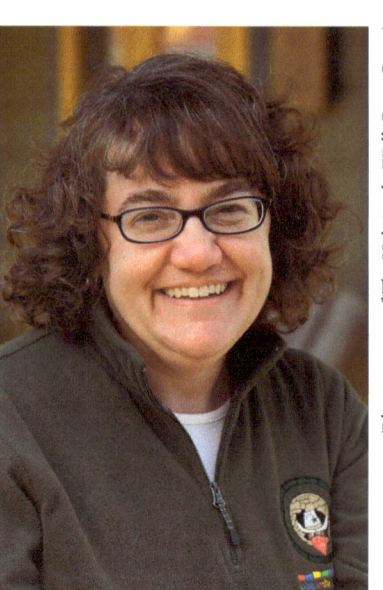

Dr. Sharon Space, Medical Director

(Photo courtesy of The Hole in the Wall Gang Camp)

Under the current medical leadership of Dr. Sharon Space, THITWGC continues providing the supportive on-site medical and nursing program necessary for children with life-threatening diseases. She recently gave me updated Camp data on milestones, campers in attendance, and their diagnoses. An overview of milestones from the medical perspective is shown in the table below to provide information on the growth in the number of sessions, the introduction of special sessions, and Camp's responses to the medical and nursing needs of campers.

Year	Milestone
1988	First summer with 4 general sessions
1989	5 sessions; first Immunology Session
1990	6 sessions; first Sickle Cell Session
1991	7 sessions; first Brother and Sister (Sibling) Session
1996	8 sessions; increased to 2 Immunology Sessions
2002	9 sessions; increased to 2 Sickle Cell Sessions
2008	First Hero's Journey sessions
2009	First planned overnight campers in the Infirmary to accommodate children with metabolic disorders needing nursing observation
2010	Decreased to 1 Immunology Session
2012	Moose Lodge opens for campers needing overnight nursing care
2013	Camp's 25th Birthday!

In 1988, there were 270 campers in attendance at general sessions; 18 of those campers came to two sessions. By 1991, we had 800 campers, a level that we maintained through 1995. During those early years, we had sessions that lasted for 11 days, except for the Sickle Cell and Brother and Sister Special Sessions that went for seven days each. Because word and positive praise had spread about THITWGC, we were receiving applications from more children than we could accommodate. Consequently, in 1996 we changed all of our sessions to seven days each to increase the service capacity. Since 2002, we have had slightly over 1,000 children each summer. Currently, we have from 110 to 140 campers during each of the nine summer sessions.

It gives me a sense of great accomplishment to reflect on the fact that from 1988 to 2014, children have had over 30,000 direct Camp experiences with us in Ashford-Eastford. In addition, there have been older teens, young adults, and families enjoying on-site Camp experiences as well as children throughout the northeastern United States benefiting from THITWGC outreach programs in hospitals.

After the first several years of Camp, the number of children attending with a diagnosis of cancer has remained between 200 and 250 each summer into the present time. These numbers reaffirm my early recommendation to Paul to include children with other life-threatening diseases beyond cancer. Sickle cell disease has had a constant presence at Camp due to early recruitment of children from Yale's clinics, the establishment of some special sessions for children with the disease, and effective recruitment through pediatric hematology clinics throughout New England. The number of campers with this diagnosis has been at over 300 each summer for over a decade. We have seen a decline in HIV/AIDS due to the improvements in diagnosis of pregnant women and subsequent treatment to virtually eliminate the vertical transmission of the disease in newborns in the United States, and we anticipate that campers with this diagnosis will soon fall below 100 per summer. In the United States and some of the Mediterranean countries, we have seen a drastic change in recent years in the prevalence of thalassemia major due to effective identification of and counseling for people with the trait. In 2014, six children with thalassemia major attended Camp;

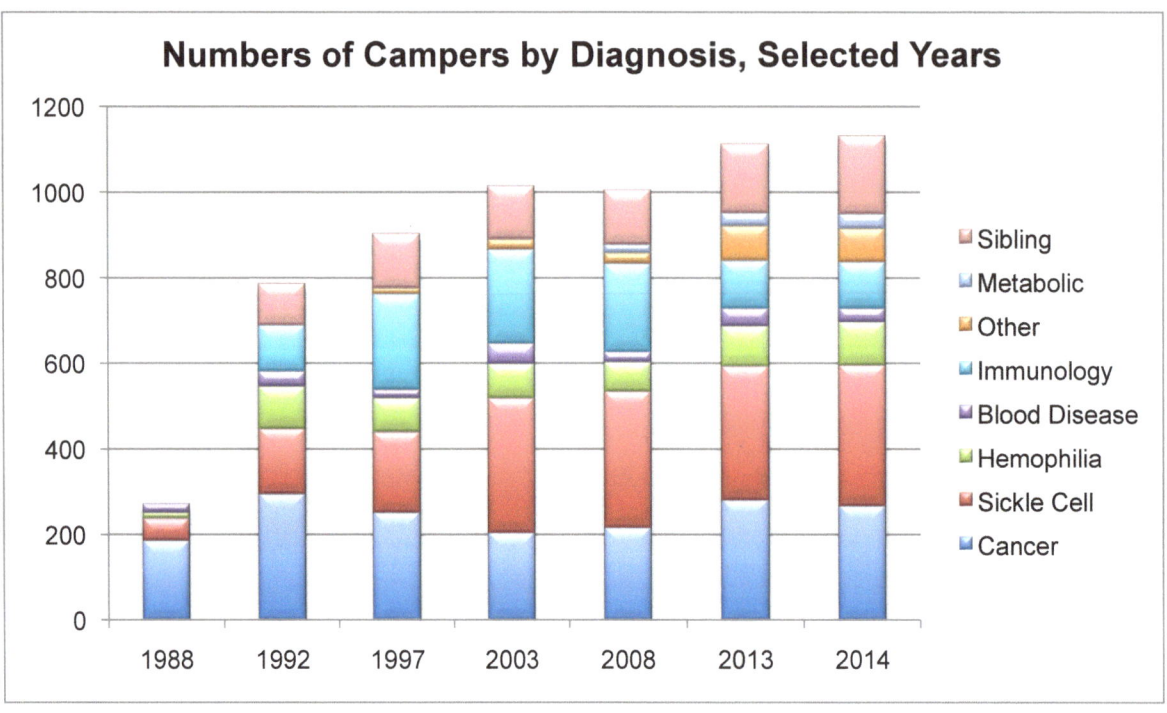

	1988	1992	1997	2003	2008	2013	2014
Siblings (healthy)	0	98	126	124	127	161	182
Other diseases	0	0	14	24	25	79	78
Metabolic diseases	0	0	0	0	20	30	35
Immunology	0	109	224	220	207	112	107
Other blood diseases	20	34	20	48	23	43	33
Hemophilia	14	99	79	81	69	94	101
Sickle cell disease	50	154	188	312	318	312	327
Cancer	186	293	251	204	215	280	267
Total campers	**270***	**798**	**892**	**1,091**	**1,055**	**1,111**	**1,130**

* Eighteen children attended twice, for a total of 288 experiences.

Infirmary Visits and Transports, Selected Years

	1988	1993	2008	2013	2014
Camper visits	1,420	2,507	1,988	2,525	2,443
Staff visits	NA	NA	589	645	386
Total visits	**1,420**	**2,507**	**2,577**	**3,170**	**2,829**
Transports	NA	5	10	10	12

NA = Not Available

and of those, five of them were of Far Eastern Asian descent. Due to Sharon's active recruitment efforts, in 2007 Camp had its first children with metabolic disorders, and the number grew to 35 in 2014. Based on my early reports to the Board and her own data collection, Sharon has provided the data and graph of camper diagnoses, shown on the opposite page.

Sharon has also provided data on Infirmary visits and transports from Camp for selected years. Because many of the staff members are former campers with medical needs that can require an Infirmary visit, Sharon began tracking those visits as well. As shown in the table on the opposite page, the volume of visits is significant during the course of a summer. In recent years, transports from Camp have averaged around ten each summer.

Some Infirmary visits involve a procedure. The most frequent procedure performed at Camp is prophylactic Factor use for boys with hemophilia. In 2014, 178 of these procedures were done at Camp, and many of them were self-administered by camper request. Overall, the medical and nursing staff and volunteers have continued to respond to the needs of campers. In 2012, the Moose Lodge was built in the area in the back of the Infirmary to accommodate campers needing overnight nursing care. While the safety of the children remains first and foremost, creative and functional ways are found to provide them with the healing experience of THITWGC.

In recent Summer Camp Evaluation Reports, Camp's Director of Research and Evaluation Ann Gillard provided carefully collected and analyzed data from campers and volunteers on their experiences and from parents on their observations of the children. Data are used to formulate Camp strengths (for example, high levels of staff attention, friendliness, and emotional safety provided by staff to campers in 2013) and look for areas that might be improved. The overwhelming majority of campers, volunteers, and parents provide immensely positive feedback through this process. Specific comments from the 2014 Evaluation Report are:

Parent quotes:
- "She said the week was life changing…taught her how to be happy again."
- "I heard, at pick up, how he really opened up and also was eager to infuse himself because his friends were doing it."
- "I love that he gets to make friends with kids, and he just doesn't 'care' why they are at Camp. Not that he doesn't care about them or their struggles, but that he doesn't let their condition define them. They are just who they are, not my friend with cancer, or my deaf friend, or my friend with sickle cell."

From volunteers:
- "A camper told me, 'At home I feel like I can't do things. Here I feel like I can do everything.'"
- "Campers were encouraged in a non-threatening way to try new things. They were allowed to participate to their maximum tolerance level and when they wanted to scale things back, it happened immediately for them. All of their accomplishments, no matter how small, were applauded."
- "A few campers who sheltered themselves and seemed withdrawn in the beginning ended up pairing with others and initiating communication and activities without staff prompting."

- "I think what struck me the most was in the Dining Hall watching everyone singing and dancing. The faces on both the campers and staff said it all. It was pure joy."

When asked what their favorite moments at Camp were, campers wrote:
- "My favorite moment at Camp was just being in the cabin with my close friends and counselors and playing all these games like silent ball and mafia. I also liked laughing and making funny jokes and everyone else laughing. I loved cabin chat because I really felt heard on my feelings and thoughts."
- "My favorite moment at Camp was Stage Night! I liked that because everyone got the courage to perform on stage, especially me."
- "My favorite moment at Camp was being able to have a normal camp experience. Also being able to meet new people with illnesses."
- "My favorite moment at Camp was seeing my cabin mates really come out of their shells and go into their stretch zones with trying new things and getting over their fears."

We see in the joyful faces of the campers what THITWGC means to them. We witness their tears when they have to leave. We know that memories, connections with Camp through the winter months, and anticipation of attending during subsequent years energize them. Dr. Richard Kayne recently related to me one of the sweetest comments I have heard by a camper: "Camp makes my heart blossom."

Once Paul was confident about our success at THITWGC, he supported efforts in the United States and around the world to serve children with serious illnesses free of charge by founding the Association of Hole in the Wall Gang Camps. Funding from Newman's Own proceeds contributed to the establishment of a series of new camps. In 2012, the name of the Association was changed to SeriousFun Children's Network. This Network continues to function, providing the members with an annual opportunity to interact and learn from each other. By 2015, there were over 600,000 children and family members served by The Hole in the Wall Gang Camp and the Network that grew out of it.[1] Anne and I had the pleasure of visiting a number of affiliated camps, including Barretstown in Ireland, Camp Boggy Creek in Florida, and The Painted Turtle in California. Mary Lou and Stephen saw the property of Victory Junction in North Carolina as land was being prepared for construction. They have visited Camp Korey in Carnation, Washington, where some of Stephen's pediatric patients have attended. While cancer remains the most common medical diagnosis that Network campers have, the different camps have included children with conditions such as gastrointestinal, rheumatological, and vascular disorders. Stephen and Mary Lou learned that Camp Korey organizes their sessions by conditions so that children referred from the Friends of Craniofacial Center or campers with skeletal dysplasia and metabolic bone conditions attend the camp with others with similar diagnoses.[2] The Network has taken Paul's dream far beyond his original idea for Connecticut.

Without a doubt, we have fulfilled Paul Newman's dream of providing a safe place "for kids to kick back, relax and raise a little hell," as the Camp motto states. I hope the future continues

---

1   www.seriousfunnetwork.org
2   campkorey.org

to bring positive change. In April 2014, I returned to Camp to participate in a staff orientation program. Ray Lamontagne, Mike Kolakowski, and I told stories about the planning, development, and early years of Camp. At one point, we were asked what we thought THITWGC might be like 50 years from now. My response was that I hoped that there would not be a need for Camp because there would be preventions and cures for the diseases that campers have. Since I began my medical career well over a half-century ago, we have made amazing progress in treating and even preventing the life-threatening diseases that affect children. I hope that progress continues or even accelerates, turning children's luck from bad to good.

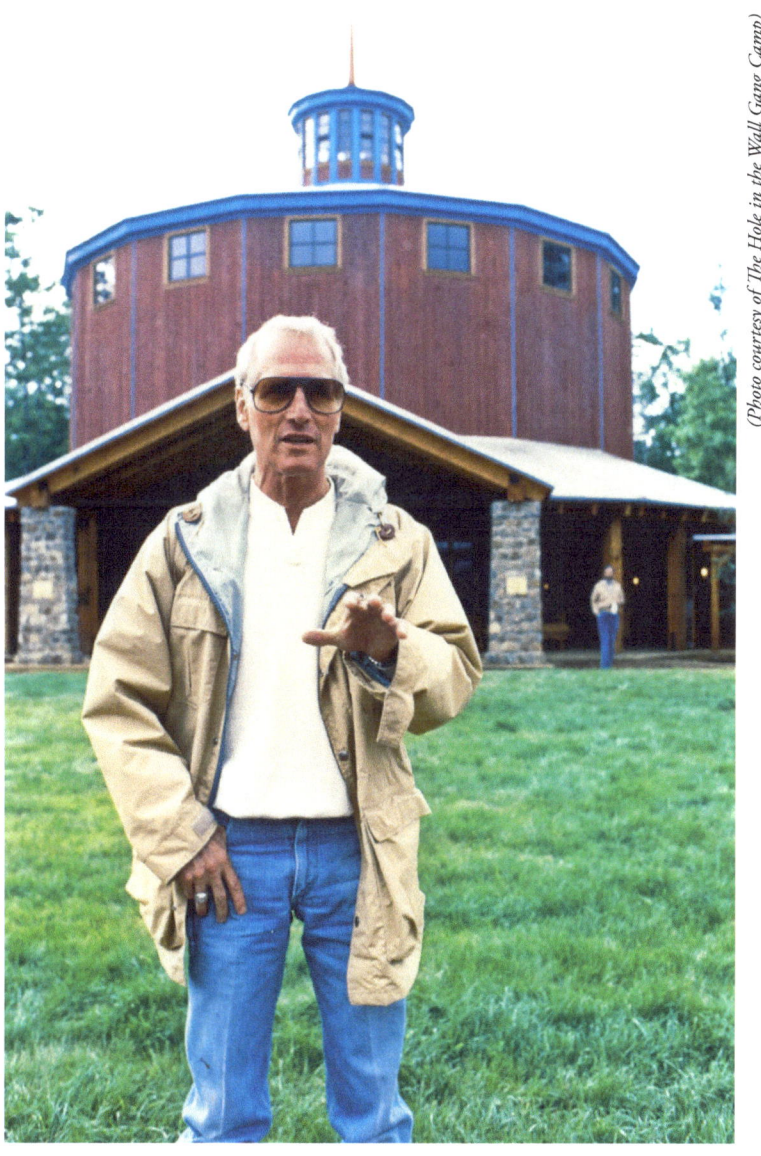

(Photo courtesy of The Hole in the Wall Gang Camp)

*I like to think that Paul is saying,
"Yes, Doctor, the dream is FULFILLED!"*

CHAPTER ELEVEN

Beyond Just a Camp Doc

My first and foremost focus during my 14 summers at THITWGC was the medical program and the safety of the children. However, I, too, was caught up in the magical fulfillment of Paul's dream. I participated in Stage Night activities as the rear end Wonky the Wonder Horse or his trainer. I dressed up as a clown to entertain children and staff. On two separate occasions during consecutive summers, I organized a cribbage tournament that was open to campers, counselors, and staff. We acquired a large, ornate trophy to create some fanfare around the competition and photo opportunities for the cribbage winner. After interested participants signed up, I arranged for play-off games. The first year, I won handily. The second year, the champion was my grandson Daniel, who was at Camp with his volunteering parents, Stephen and Mary Lou. Years later, Dan's essay in his MD/PhD applications included a poignant section on his experiences at Camp that motivated him to pursue medicine as a career. He currently attends Harvard Medical School.

As a clown

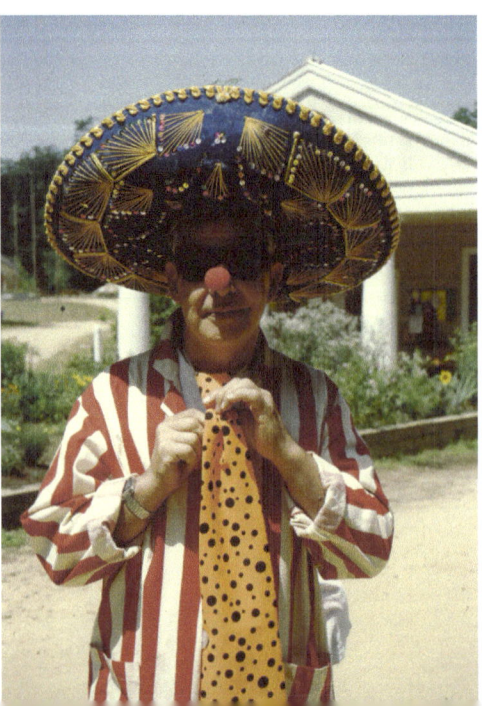

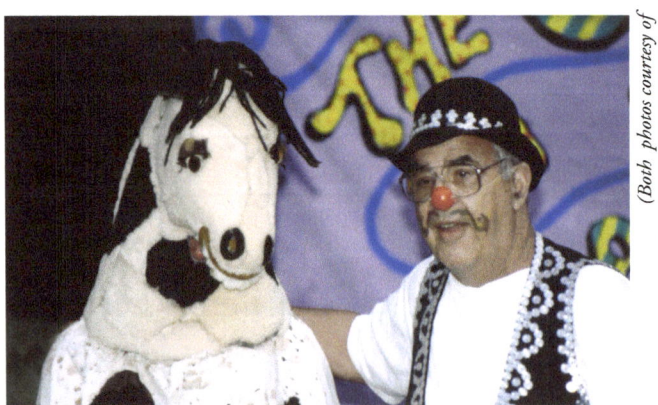

Wonky on stage, with me as his trainer

(Both photos courtesy of The Hole in the Wall Gang Camp)

I also wrote a song for Camp: **Doc's Camp Song**

Oh, won't you come back to our Camp, it's the best Camp in the land.
Where there's swimming and hiking, and the food is oh so grand.
There may be others, but brothers, they just don't compare.
And when you come back to our Camp,
We'll be waiting for you there.
Oh, won't you come back to our Camp, it's the best Camp that's around,
Where there's singing and dancing, and the couns-lors never frown.
There may be others, but brothers, we'll stay for a while,
Oh, won't you come back to our Camp where the campers wear a -
They're never frowning,
Where the campers wear a -
They're always grinning,
Where the campers wear a SMILE.

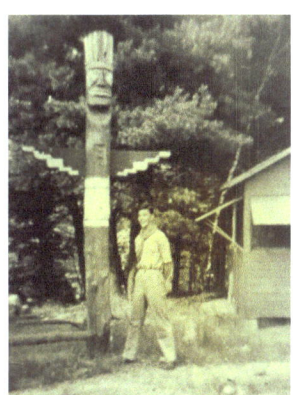

With my first totem pole in 1944

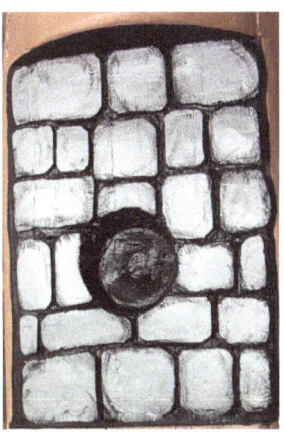

Hole in the Wall totem

But perhaps my most interesting activity at Camp was carving the totem poles. As a Native American cultural and artistic tradition in the Pacific Northwest, totem poles are a collection of symbols (totems) of kinship, legends, significant people, and notable events carved into large red cedar logs and painted. They can serve to identify a clan or family.

During the construction of THITWGC in 1987-88, I thought about creating a totem pole to capture the meaning and spirit of Camp that was unfolding and add to the Western motif so desired by Paul. In 1944, at the Boy Scout's Camp Powow near Amesbury, Massachusetts, I had carved a totem pole as my Eagle Scout project. Early in 1988, I made a preliminary sketch of the first totem pole on Yale-New Haven Hospital stationary and named the pole "PROMISE." As I planned it, I wrote a legend to describe it.

Between 1988 and 2008, I designed and carved nine totem poles to capture the spirit and magic of this special place for children with cancer and other life-threatening diseases. These poles, along with their legends and explanations of the totems, are presented here.

The poles have some recurrent themes that are depicted through totems conveying the spirit of Camp. The most frequent theme is a stone wall with a hole in its middle, literally the "The Hole in the Wall," representing the name chosen by Paul for its symbolism as a refuge from illness that Camp offers. The hole in the wall symbol is carved on the all of totem poles except for WHIMSY (1993).

The Little Bandit represents the children at Camp and is carved on the 1992, '93, '94, and '96 poles. The figure was originally sketched

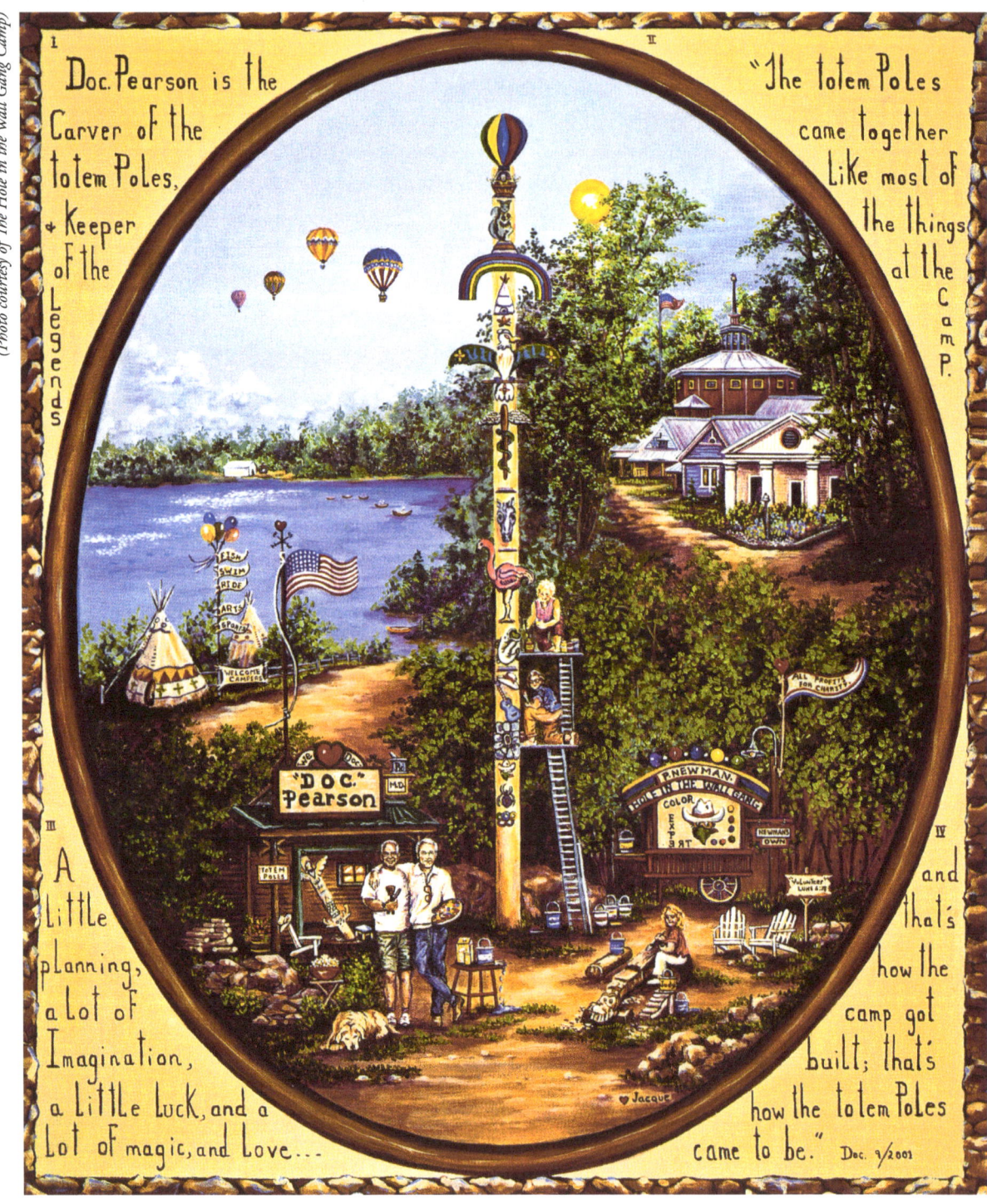

Doc Pearson, Carver of the Totem Poles
*This photo is of an original painting presented to Camp in 2003 by artist Jacqué Baker.
The 1996 totem pole of OLYMPICS is featured. Sherry Talley and my wife Anne are
in the scaffolding repainting a pole, and Alice Trillin is painting another pole on the ground.
Jacqué's artwork portrays a touching composite of sites around the Camp.*

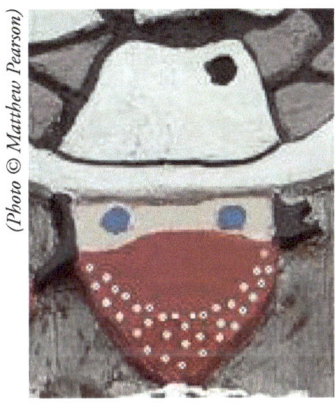

Little Bandit, 1994

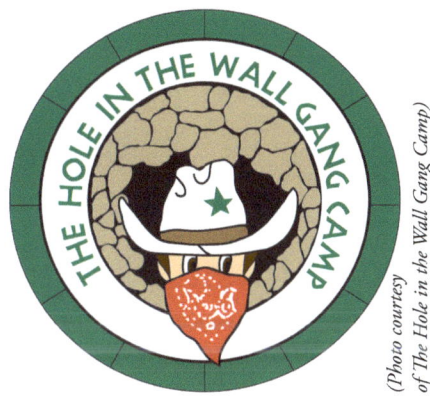

Camp logo

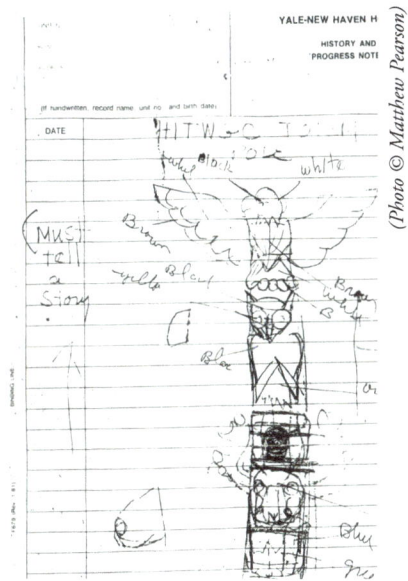

Preliminary sketch of PROMISE

by Andrea Padula and became Camp's logo.

Paul Newman is variously represented on four totem poles. A moose appears on the first one as a tribute to him and is referred to as Paul NewMoose. In the first session in 1988, Paul joined campers and staff in the Dining Hall. A camper, who probably did not know who Paul was, snatched the expensive, broad-brimmed Stetson hat that he was wearing and flipped it into the air. It landed on the antler of an antique stuffed moose mounted on the wall. That moose became known as "Paul NewMoose." Periodically thereafter, whatever hat Paul wore into the Dining Hall would be snatched and tossed up onto the moose antlers. The moose on the first pole in 1988 has vivid blue eyes, made with reflectors, as close as possible to the color of Paul's eyes.

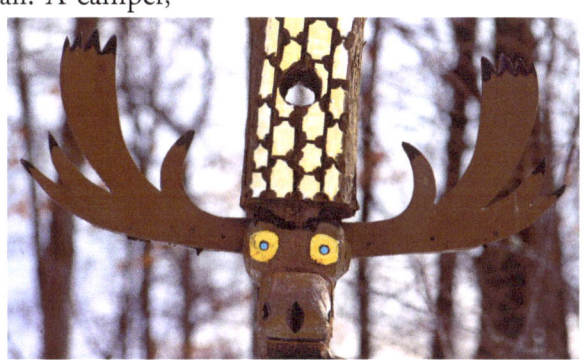

Paul NewMoose, 1988

On the 1993 pole named WHIMSY, the skunk (or polecat) with blue eyes represents PaulCat. I came up with the idea of using a skunk, which is also known as a polecat, for a whimsy, double meaning to represent PaulCat. One day when Paul was visiting Camp, he stopped by as Anne was painting the skunk. She told him that a skunk is also called a polecat, which is close to PaulCat. She pointed out the bright blue eyes she had just

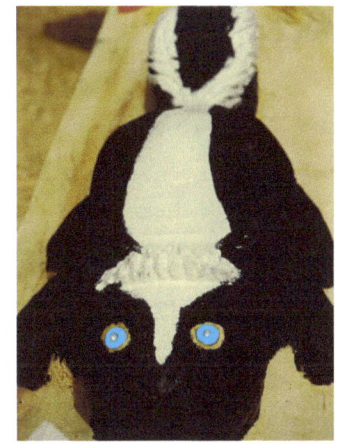

Skunk/polecat/PaulCat

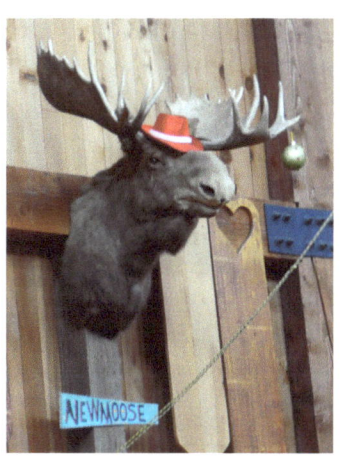

Paul NewMoose mounted on Dining Hall wall

CHAPTER 11 - Beyond Just a Camp Doc

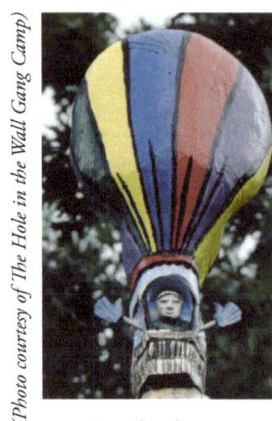

(Photo courtesy of The Hole in the Wall Gang Camp)

Paul piloting a hot air balloon, 1996

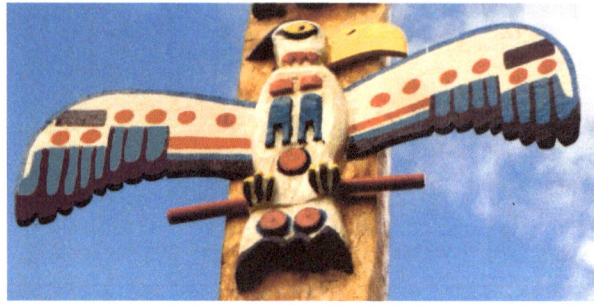

Thunderbird, 1994

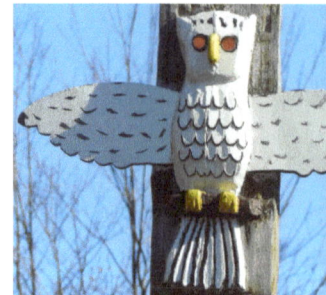

Great horned owl, 1994

painted. Paul just smiled. We think he was pleased, just as he was with the NewMoose totem.

Paul NewMoose appears again but with real antlers on the 1994 pole (see page 94). Male moose shed their antlers from December to February in the U.S., and they can be found in forests and woods. Again, the eyes of the moose were painted a vivid blue. Paul appears for the fourth time on OLYMPICS, the 1996 totem pole, as the aviator in the hot air balloon.

Thunderbirds, with wide-spreading ornate wings and prominent yellow beaks, are present on five totem poles. The thunderbird was a Native American totem signifying the connections and communications between the Earth and the Heavens. With its wide wingspan, the thunderbird carries the voices and laughter of the campers into the sky.

I carved owls on three totem poles. The first one was a barn owl (1988), the second was a snowy owl (1989), and the third was a great horned owl (1994). Perhaps because of their intense eyes, owls have been a symbol of wisdom since ancient times. They signify the special wisdom that children at Camp share with each other and their ability to see through the darkness and into the light.

Leaves of the American chestnut tree are depicted on the 1989 and 1994 poles. Before 1904, the chestnut was a predominant tree in the great forests where Camp is today. Then, a fungal disease called chestnut blight infected the trees, destroying all of them in two short decades. But because the rootstocks were not killed, they periodically send up new shoots with leaves. However, these shoots grow only a little before the still-present fungus causes them to die. But they keep trying to grow, again and again. The chestnut leaves on the poles are symbols of determination, courage, survival, and rebirth. The Hole in the Wall Gang Camp is a rootstalk for our children. They keep on trying to grow up.

As the first totem pole began taking shape, the process for creating them became apparent. After 1988, I sketched the designs directly on the logs. To carve, chip, and shape, I used a wooden mallet and wood chisels. For deep cuts, I enlisted George Harakaly, who used his chain saw. I joked that it was a "Native American" chain saw because I wanted the process to follow Native carving traditions. The holes in the Hole in the Wall totems were all made by George with his so-called Native American chain saw. My final task prior to painting was sanding the totems, which I did with an electrical sander and referred to it as my "Aboriginal sander."

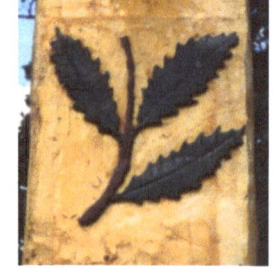

Chestnut leaves, 1994

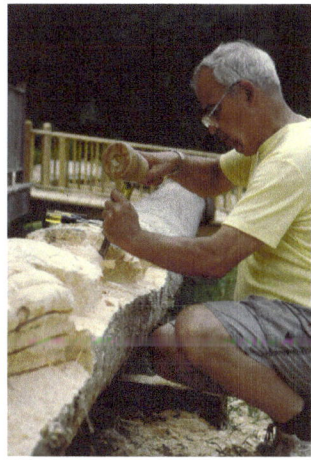 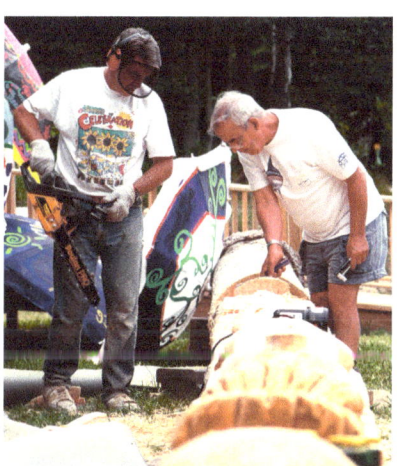 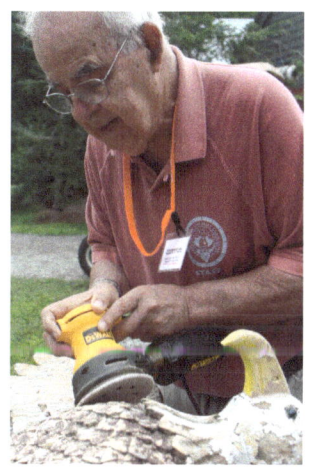

Using a wooden mallet   *With George and his Native American Chain Saw*   *Using my "Aboriginal sander"*

At times, volunteers and staff would help me.

I carved all of the poles in an open area between the Wood Shop and the Infirmary because I needed convenient access to woodworking tools while also being available at the Infirmary in a moment's notice. The carving became a diversion to keep me busy while always ready to see an ill child.

Although most of the totems were cut directly into the logs, appendages were needed to create some figures. These included the wings of the pink pig, as well as the wings and beaks of the various birds, the horns of the buffalo, the elephant ears and tusks, the tail of the wolf, one set of moose antlers, the snouts of some of the animals, the front paws of the bears and beaver, and the flamingo neck and tail.

Most of the appendages were made in the Wood Shop using a band saw to cut wood into these shapes. When it came to using electric saws, I asked for help from the Wood Shop staff to avoid cutting my own fingers. Frank Meduna, a worker in Maintenance, became my "appendage man" for many of the totems.

My brother Buddy, a carpenter, and his brother-in-law artist Armand Sindoni visited Camp while the first totem pole was being carved in 1988. Armand was a close friend of mine in high school. Buddy and Armand were the first of many friends and family who

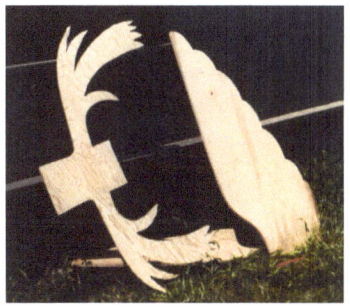 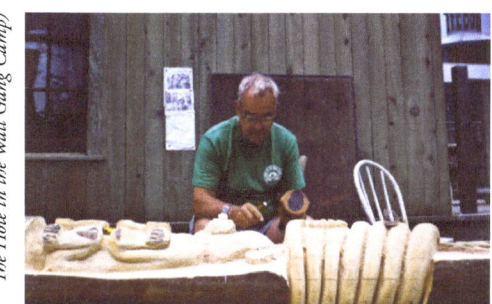 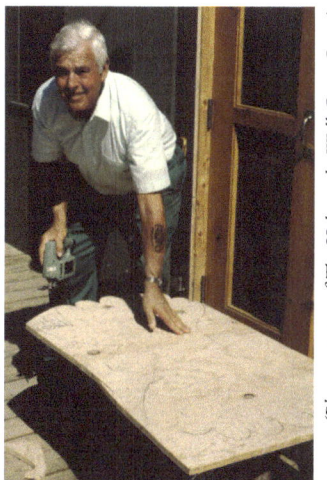

Moose antlers and eagle wing appendages, 1988   *Carving behind the Wood Shop and Infirmary, with the Dining Hall in the background at the right*   *My brother Buddy plying his carpentry skills*

visited me over the years at Camp and often lent a hand to work on a totem pole. Buddy cut the plywood for the eagle wings and moose antlers.

Campers were involved in the process by offering comments, suggestions, and encouragement. The central location of the carving site allowed ample opportunities for the children, the counselors, and the volunteers to see the process and talk with me outside of the Infirmary/medical setting.

Although many people participated in the painting, my main painters were Sherry Talley and Anne. While I had some suggestions for colors, I gave them both artistic license to select the colorful paints that would bring vibrancy to each totem.

The Maintenance Crew was usually responsible for digging the holes, but occasionally I helped. Paul also contributed. His job was to paint with tar the butt ends of the poles that go into the ground. He insisted that this would help preserve them. When a totem pole was completed and the hole was ready, George and the Maintenance Crew would transport it to its planting site using a tractor with an arm. The butt end was placed in the hole, the pole was lifted vertically with pulleys and ropes, and the base was set with firmly packed dirt, sometimes supervised by Paul.

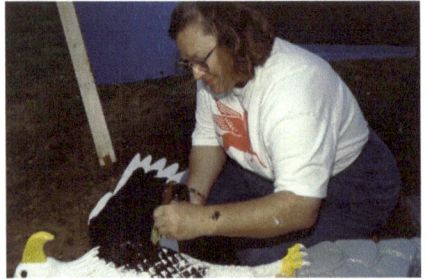

Sherry painting the eagle on the top of VIGILANCE, 1994

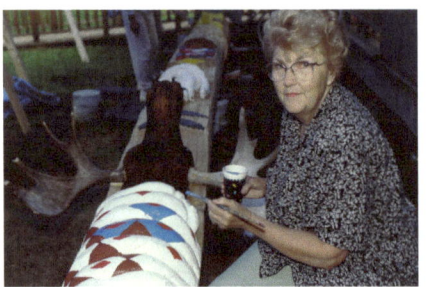

Anne painting a colorful snake

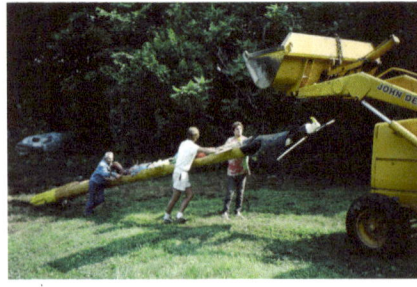

Moving the heavy VIGILANCE from the carving to its planting site near Camp's entrance

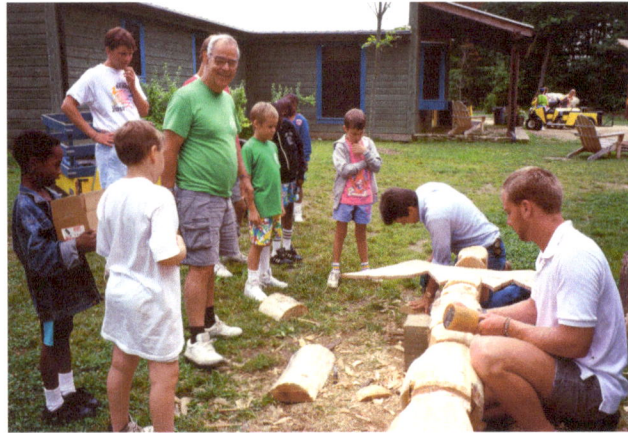

Campers watching the carving and commenting, 1990

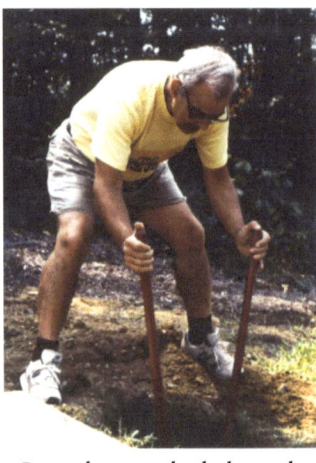

I am digging the hole in the ground for PROMISE, 1988

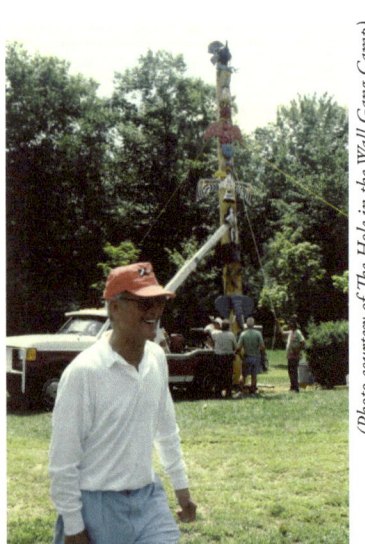

Paul at the planting of WHIMSY, 1993

The Legend of PROMISE, 1988

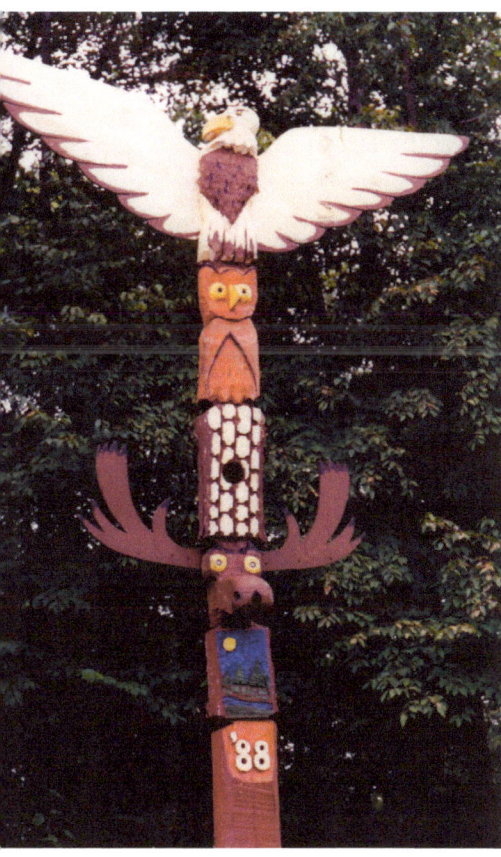

In the beginning, there were the WOODS.
Tall green pine, and oak and maple.
And there were WATERS, blue and dancing in the SUN.

But the WOODS and WATERS were silent,
For nowhere could be heard the voices
and the laughter of the children.

And the spirit of the GREAT NEWMOOSE
came to the land,
And he had a dream and vision of what might be;

And he built THE HOLE IN THE WALL GANG CAMP.

And the children, special brave children,
came to Camp in ever larger numbers.
Living and playing together,
they gained a special WISDOM of themselves and each other.

And they left these WOODS and WATERS, this Camp,
with a soaring spirit of FREEDOM
and a wider VISION of their lives and of the future.

PROMISE
(Photo courtesy of The Hole in the Wall Gang Camp)

PROMISE was carved in the summer of 1988, the first year of THITWGC. For this pole, I used a 30-foot tall hickory log that had been felled during Camp construction the year before. Three additional totem poles would be made from trees cut down during construction.

With all of the other totem poles, I started carving at the top and finished at the bottom, planning the figures and their legends as I worked down the log. In 1988, I wrongly thought that the story related by a totem pole should be read from the bottom up, not from the top down, so PROMISE might be considered upside down! To be consistent with the 1988 legend as I originally wrote it, the totems for PROMISE will be explained beginning at the bottom. The subsequent totem poles are read beginning at the top and going down.

The totem above '88 acknowledges the woods in northeast Connecticut where Camp was built—land with blue calming waters, as well as pine, oak, and maple trees. Sunny days make the skies a deep azure and Pearson Pond a shining, glimmering blue.

Going up the pole are Paul NewMoose, the hole in the wall, and the orange barn owl, all of which were explained as recurrent themes. The eagle at the top of "PROMISE" appears with wings ready for soaring with a new sense of freedom and independence that the children gain from Camp.

CHAPTER 11 ~ Beyond Just a Camp Doc

The carving of PROMISE took most of the first summer. After painting was completed during the last Camp session in August, the pole was planted on the edge of the green, facing the Dining Hall, and covered with a blue tarp. On the last evening of the last session in 1988 after the Awards Night Program in the Gymnasium, the children walked in the dark along a candlelit path to PROMISE. I unveiled the first totem pole and told its legend to the children. Two weeks later, Paul attached a plaque to the pole and formally dedicated it to the first counselors and staff.

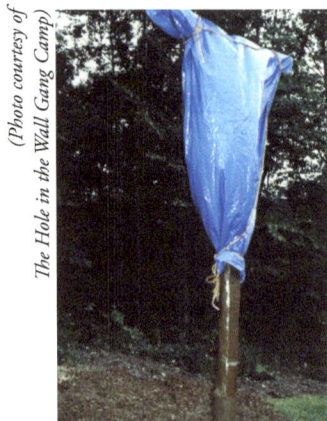

PROMISE, covered with a blue tarp, awaiting the unveiling

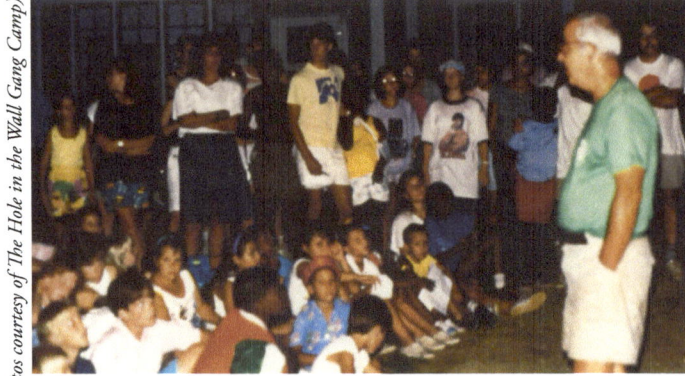

Relating the legend of PROMISE to campers

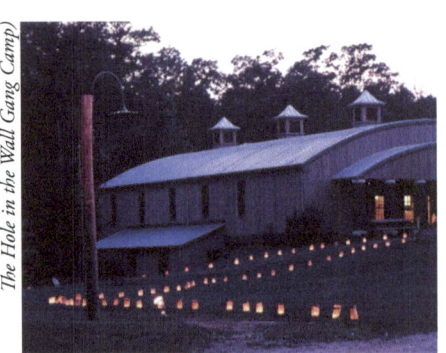

The candlelit path from the Gymnasium

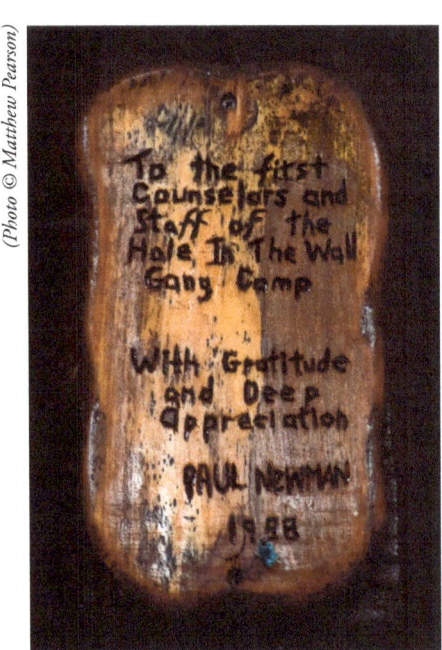

Paul's plaque

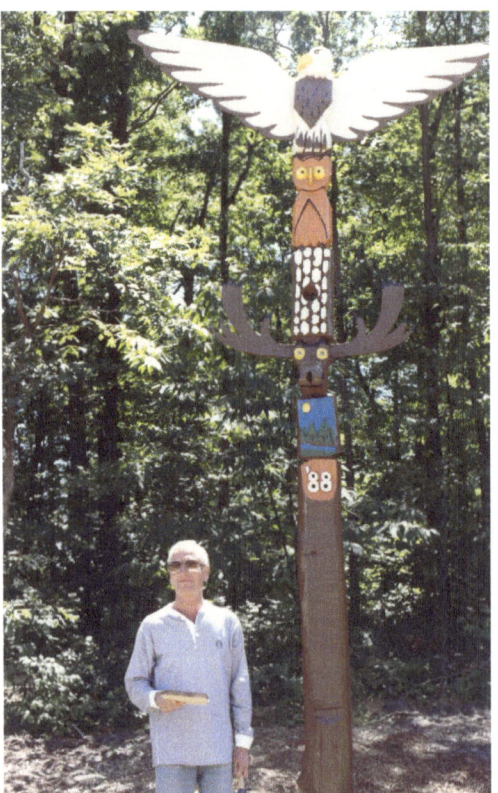

Paul dedicating PROMISE

The Legend of HOPE, 1989

What is this Camp?

*It is the dignity and the independence of the BUFFALO
that once roamed the wide plains in countless millions.*

*It is the wile and strength of the great FISH
that swims the depths of the blue waters,
and not only survives, but prevails.*

*It is the vision and wisdom of the SNOWY OWL
that is able to see through the darkness
and into the dawn.*

*It is the determination and courage
of the AMERICAN CHESTNUT –
a tree that a century ago dominated the forests of Camp.
Cut to its rootstalk by a savage blight, it still endures,
sending branches and leaves into the sky, again and yet again.*

*What is Camp?
It is all of these.
For these are the CHILDREN.
They are THE HOLE IN THE WALL GANG CAMP.*

HOPE

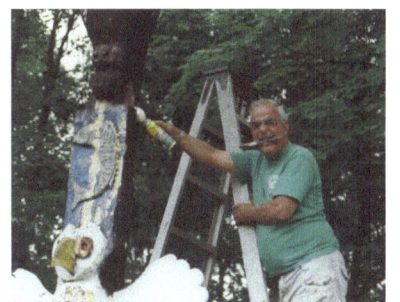

Using putty in a futile attempt to repair the termite-eaten buffalo head and fish

It turns out that if you do anything once at Camp, it can become a tradition. When Camp opened for the second season, I was repeatedly asked, "When are you going to start another totem pole?" I decided to carve a second one using an oak log that had a big knob on its top that I carved into a buffalo head.

At some early point, the legend of Wee-Pee, an enormous mythical fish, spread among the campers, prompting me to carve him below the buffalo on the totem pole. Wee-Pee is the big legendary fish in Pearson Pond that has never been seen, but everybody wants to catch!

After only a few years, we realized that because the logs used for some of the early totem poles had lain on the ground, they had become infested with termites. Despite Paul's painting of their ends with tar, they began to disintegrate. HOPE was one of those. It was made from a red oak log that had lain on the ground since before Camp construction began in 1987, and it was reduced to a pile of sawdust by termites with help from woodpeckers. Only the owl's beak and wings and the horns of the buffalo remained. The 1989 totem pole survives only in photographs.

CHAPTER 11 ~ *Beyond Just a Camp Doc*

The Legend of CREATION, 1990

*The GREAT SPIRIT wanted to build a camp
for a special group of courageous children
and brought together his animal friends for counsel.*

*The BLACK RAVEN advised,
"The Camp must be open to the sky, sun, and stars,
so the children's spirits can soar
and know what it is to be free."*

*The GRAY WOLF counseled,
"The Camp must have deep green woods with long paths
through which the children can run
and learn the hidden secrets and surprises of nature."*

*The BROWN BEAR laughed,
"The Camp must have warm and cozy places
where the children can live and play
and learn from each other."*

*And the voices of the ANCIENT INDIANS
rose from this land where they had lived and hunted
so long ago.*

*Their murmurs were heard by the GREAT SPIRIT
and He knew where Camp would be built.*

*And He threw a mighty LIGHTNING BOLT
to mark this place –
THE HOLE IN THE WALL GANG CAMP.*

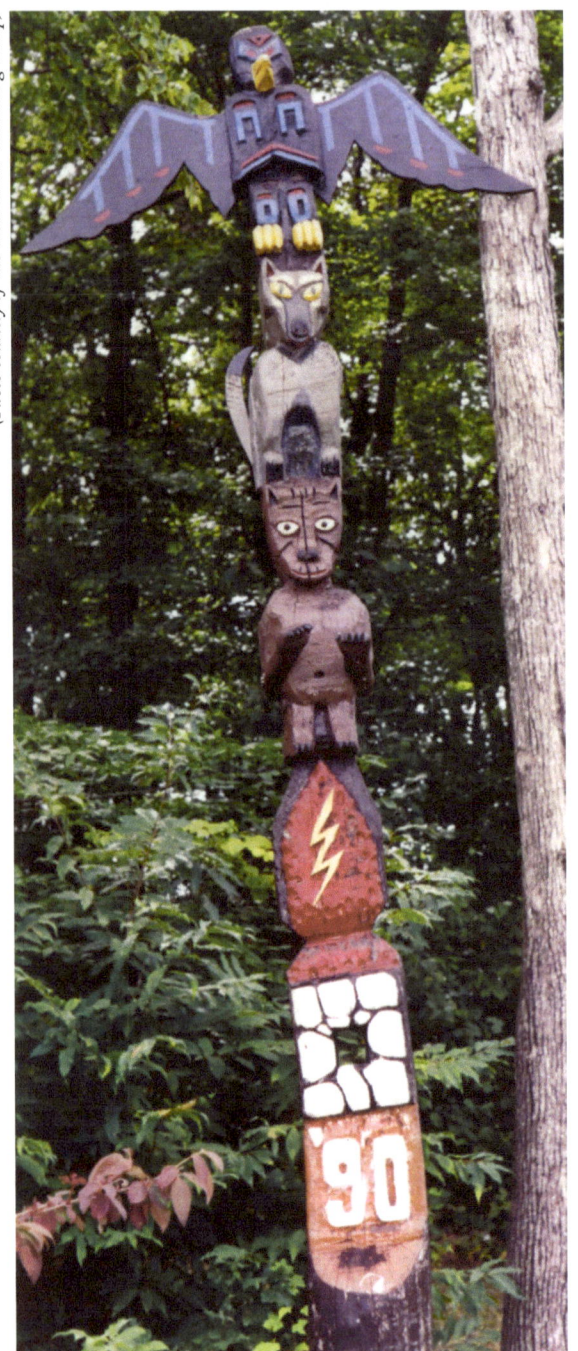

(Photo courtesy of The Hole in the Wall Gang Camp)

CREATION

In the third summer of THITWGC, another felled hickory log was chosen to carve CREATION that told yet another legend of Camp's beginning, leaning heavily on the traditions and symbols of Native Americans.

To tell the story of how Camp came to be, I began with a black raven, with wide wings for soaring in the sky and a sense of freedom that we want to convey to campers. The raven, closely related to the crow family, reminds me of George's tame crow named Jeremiah, who enjoyed perching on the shoulders of campers and staff. He was a friendly, inquisitive bird who flew freely around his chosen home at Camp.

Below the raven is a gray wolf, who told the Great Spirit that paths through the woods were needed at Camp. The gray wolf acknowledges the Connecticut U.S. Naval Reserve Construction Battalion volunteers who built the bridges over the wetlands and paths through the woods during their two weeks of active duty in the spring of 1988.

Next is a brown bear, who wanted warm, cozy places. Camp has them—the cabins, all of the facilities, and the overall environment are welcoming, comfortable, and comforting.

The lightening bolt symbolizes the Great Spirit's selection of the land for Camp. It might also give an indication of the speed at which Camp was built! The arrowhead, on which it is displayed, acknowledges the Native people of the land. Finishing off the pole are the recurrent themes of the hole in the wall and the year. After several years outdoors, CREATION was placed in the Dining Hall for safekeeping.

After carving the first three poles, I selected and recreated four of their totems to adorn the podium used in the Dining Hall: Paul NewMoose, the lightning bolt on an arrowhead, the hole in the wall, and the chestnut leaves. They capture Camp's spirit and provide color to the otherwise plain podium.

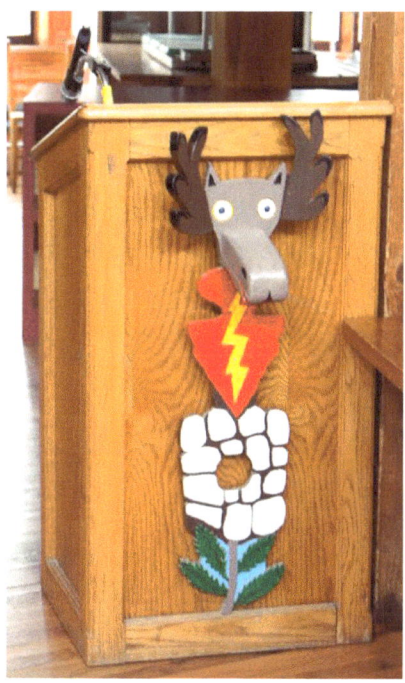

Recreated totems on the podium in the Dining Hall

CHAPTER 11 ~ Beyond Just a Camp Doc

(Photo courtesy of The Hole in the Wall Gang Camp)

SPIRIT – the original

The Legend of SPIRIT, 1991

The THUNDERBIRD,
carrier of the voices and the laughter
from the children to the Great Spirit on high.

The TURTLE,
whose shell reflects the round globe of the earth.

The BEAVER,
symbolic of how man lives with
but only gently modifies nature for his needs,
as well as the busy-ness of the campers.

The FROG that represents the waters –
the good rain, the pond,
and the campers' tears of both sorrow and joy.

The INDIAN who is Camp,
his feathers are the colors of the Camp Units.

In the summer of 1991, I carved SPIRIT. Unfortunately, it was also made from a log infested with termites. As deterioration began, woodpeckers attacked it with their hollow peck-peck-peck sounds. The thunderbird, turtle, and beaver were lost. The remaining pole with a newly carved thunderbird on top was relocated to the Dining Hall.

On the original pole, the turtle, whose round shell represents the Earth, was underneath the thunderbird with its head tucked between the bird's talons.

The beaver symbolized interactions with nature, as well as the busy-ness of the children—a camper is "as busy as a beaver." The beaver was holding and gnawing on a log taken from a beaver dam down the road from Camp. The log had real teeth marks, evidence that a gnawing beaver had prepared it for the dam.

To include some of the nature around

Camp and to represent water, I carved a frog that spends part of its life in water. I used golf balls for the frog's eyes, but I would tell the children that they were really "ocular prostheses!"

Beneath the frog is a fishing fly, inspired by volunteer Tom Earnheart. As mentioned previously, Tom initiated "Save the Worm Week" and taught campers how to make fishing flies.

The land of Camp was originally occupied by indigenous tribes, and I honored them with the Indian. His eyes are carved so that they follow you when you cross in front of him. The feathers in the headdress are the colors of the Camp Units. The six feathers include the original white color of the Unit and its replacement color of purple.

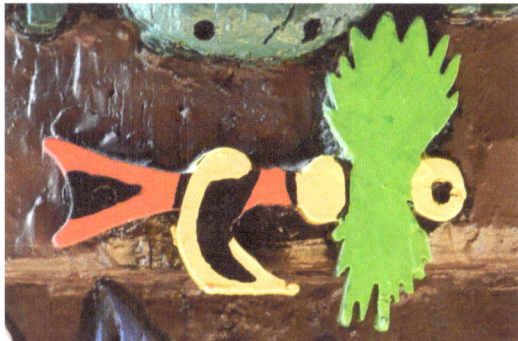

Fishing fly

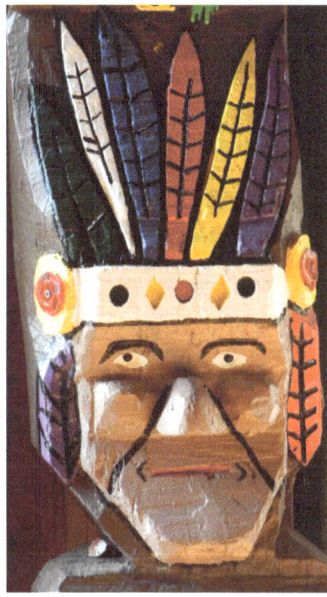

In honor of indigenous tribes

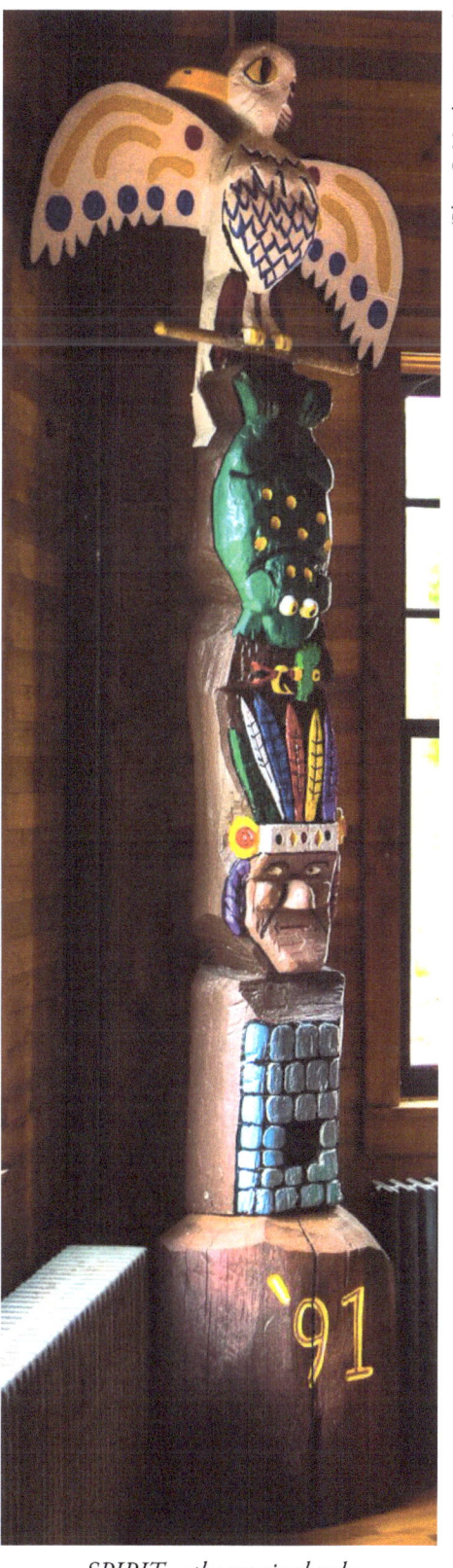

SPIRIT – the repaired pole in the Dining Hall

CHAPTER 11 ~ *Beyond Just a Camp Doc*

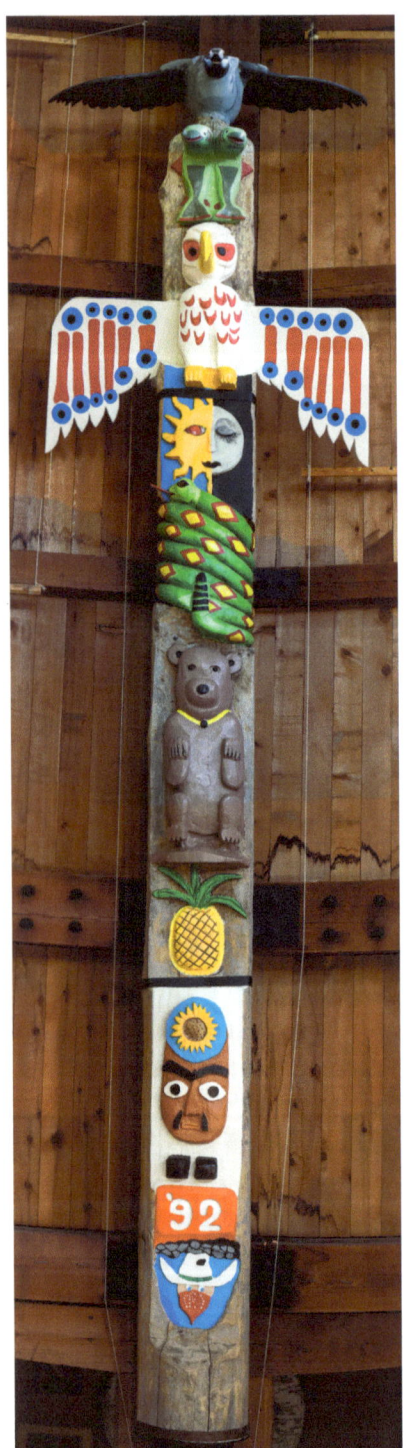

FULFILLMENT

(Photo © Matthew Pearson)

The Legend of FULFILLMENT, 1992
"The Fulfilled Dream"

*Camp is CANADA GOOSE that has her goslings at Camp,
and after summer sends them into the wide world,
stronger and more confident.*

*Camp is FISH and WATER;
the WATERS of the pond and streams,
but also the tears of the campers –
tears of both joy and sorrow.*

*Camp is THUNDERBIRD
that the Indians believed carried voices and laughter
between the Earth and the Heavens.*

*Camp is SUN-MOON;
DAY-NIGHT;
HAPPINESS-SORROW.*

*Camp is the GREAT SNAKE
that is danger but also healing.*

*The BROWN BEAR
that is power, but also protection.*

*The PINEAPPLE
that is welcome and acceptance.*

*But most of all,
Camp is the CHILDREN and the adults they will become—
GIRL-WOMAN, BOY-MAN.
The CHILDREN who have been and will be
enriched and strengthened by Camp, now and in the future.*

In the winter of 1991-92, Paul asked repeatedly, "When are you going to start another pole?" When I told him I did not have a good log, he asked what I needed. I replied, "A small red cedar log like the Northwest Native Americans used would be easy to carve and resistant to termites and rot." Within a month, a 50-foot yellow cedar log—the kind used for pencils—was delivered from the West Coast. As we started our fifth summer, I was confident that we had successfully reached the fulfillment of

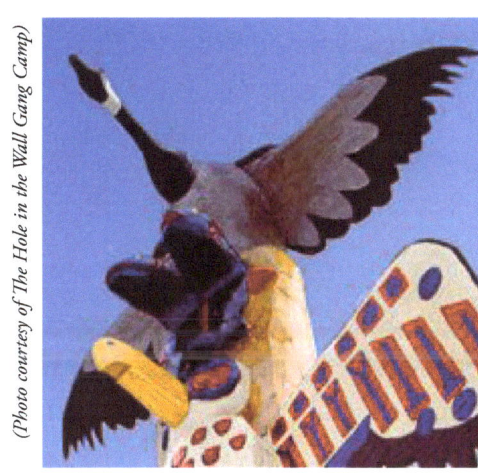
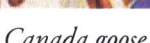

Canada goose

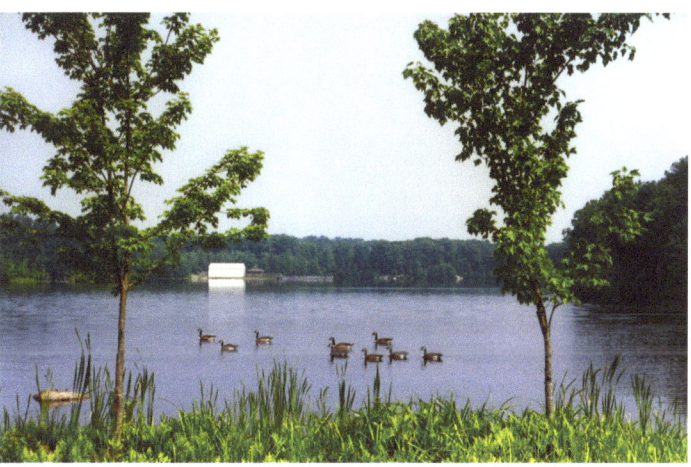

Canada geese on Pearson Pond

Paul's dream. This large log became FULFILLMENT. THITWGC fulfills Paul's dream year after year, and this book is named to celebrate the continued fulfillment of his dream.

FULFILLMENT has a Canada goose at the top because geese are often seen at Camp, either soaring in the sky or swimming. After the pole was completed and planted in the ground, the goose's neck broke off. Although I reattached it, the angle changed a bit. The original bird was looking toward the skies, while the repaired one is glancing downward at Camp.

Below FULFILLMENT's goose are two fish. These fish do not represent Wee-Pee, who is one-of–a-kind. Instead, they symbolize all of the other fish that swim in Pearson Pond that the children catch and throw back.

The sun-moon is one of my favorite totems because of the mixture of contrast and emotions it depicts, reflective of the reality of Camp—day and night, joy and sorrow.

Appearing on a pole for the first time, the snake is a symbol of both the danger of disease and treatments. There is a parallel with the snake's poison and treatment with chemotherapy, which in the right dosage can kill cancer cells but spare the healthy cells.

The brown bear below the snake is not the fuzzy bear carved into the 1990 totem pole. Instead, this one is somewhat of a paradox, representing danger but also power and protection, which is what we try to provide for the children at THITWGC.

Next is a bright yellow-orange pineapple. As a traditional symbol of welcoming associated with the return of sailing ships during the 18th century, the pineapple signifies that Camp is a welcoming place.

Below the pineapple, a "girl-woman, boy-man" figure with a sunflower on the head is an amalgamation of the campers and the adults they will become. The sunflower, which also appears on the last totem pole (OMEGA), can be seen throughout Camp in the summer when they blossom. Sue Wheeler, a volunteer who does our gardening, plants sunflowers every year with seeds supplied by her dear friend Valerie.

CHAPTER 11 ~ *Beyond Just a Camp Doc*

The Legend of WHIMSY, 1993

*The TURKEY is a noble bird to be sure,
but whimsy says that other kinds of turkeys have been at Camp.*

*The CRICKET and LADY BUG
with their HARVEST of good luck.*

*Who ever saw a PINK PIG WITH WINGS
sitting on top of the WORLD?
At Camp, why not?*

*A RAINBOW FISH jumping over a THUNDERBIRD.
At Camp it could happen.*

*The SKUNK, also called POLECAT,
with blue eyes at that.
Whimsy says that it was PAULCAT
who made Camp happen.*

*The SUN that shines over the SENTINEL TREE
even when it rains.*

*The GENTLE DEER
that guard Camp when the children leave.*

*The ELEPHANTS who came
and captured Camp and the children's hearts.*

*Whimsy can only be a breath away from heartbreak at Camp.
The 1993 totem pole is for our littlest PICKLE-EATER.
We miss you, Melissa.*

WHIMSY, defined as a capricious and fanciful creation, was a theme at THITWGC during the summer of 1993. This totem pole does not tell a single story but has many legends for those of us who have been privileged to live and work in this special place.

On top is a wild turkey, which can be found in rural areas around New England. Traditionally prepared for Thanksgiving dinners, they are fun birds to watch but a challenge to carve! Frank Meduna, the appendage man, created the more difficult

(Photo © Matthew Pearson)

WHIMSY

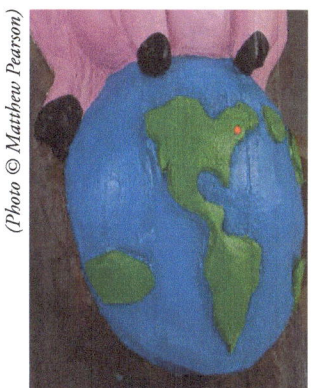

Fanciful, whimsical, winged pink pig, inspired by Betty

The red dot marks Camp!

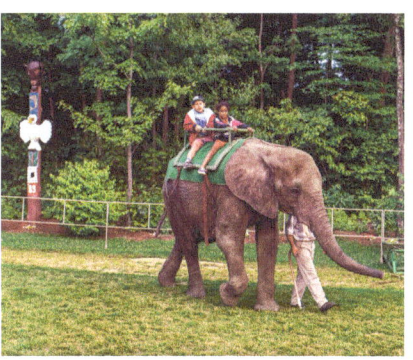

Elephants came to give rides to campers!

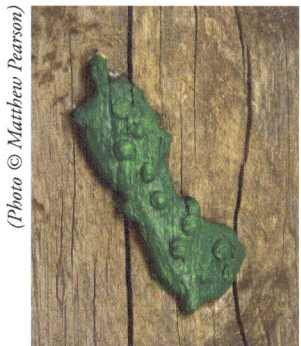

A pickle for Melissa

pieces—the tail feathers and wings—by piecing together individual strips of wood. The double meanings of some of the totems on this pole start with the turkey as noble, yet, sometimes a bit foolish.

The cricket, sheaved wheat, and ladybug in a three-in-one totem below the turkey represent a harvest of good luck. We want lots of good luck at Camp! A cricket is also found on the very top of the Dining Hall in the form of a weather vane.

Why did I carve a pink pig with wings on the pole? Betty, the Vietnamese pot-bellied pig brought to Camp by Dr. Sam Ross, inspired this totem. On the globe underneath the pink pig is a red spot marking the location of Camp in North America. At Camp, we sometimes feel that we are sitting on top of the world just like the pink pig!

Above the recurrent thunderbird is a jumping rainbow fish. Thunderbirds are likely to eat fish, not let them jump over their heads. The seemingly impossible fish and thunderbird relationship is pure whimsy.

Below the skunk (polecat, for PaulCat), is the Sentinel Tree on the sun. This represents the pine tree on the edge of Pearson Pond named by Mary Harper, the Camp Archivist for many years. She said it "watched as Camp was being built." With a beaming sun as the backdrop, the Tree represents the beauty of THITWGC.

Below the Sentinel Tree is a deer that was carved by Woody, Camp Director at the time. The deer in the region are plentiful, coming out at after dark and disappearing with the sunrise. The antlers on this pole were found on Camp property and were used as a natural appendage. Male deer grow and shed new antlers every year.

Although they came for only one Camp session, the elephants were magnificent and magical. Someone who had elephants had heard about THITWGC and offered to bring them on site. The children were able to ride on these intelligent and empathetic animals. Paul and I got rides, too. We all loved it! The Little Bandit, cuddled in the elephant's trunk, is a repeating theme representing the campers.

The last totem on this pole is a pickle, perhaps the only one ever to be carved on a totem pole. This special totem represents our pickle-eater Little Melissa, a child who came to Camp for several summers. She would only eat pickles. Melissa had passed away from her disease during the wintertime.

CHAPTER 11 ~ Beyond Just a Camp Doc

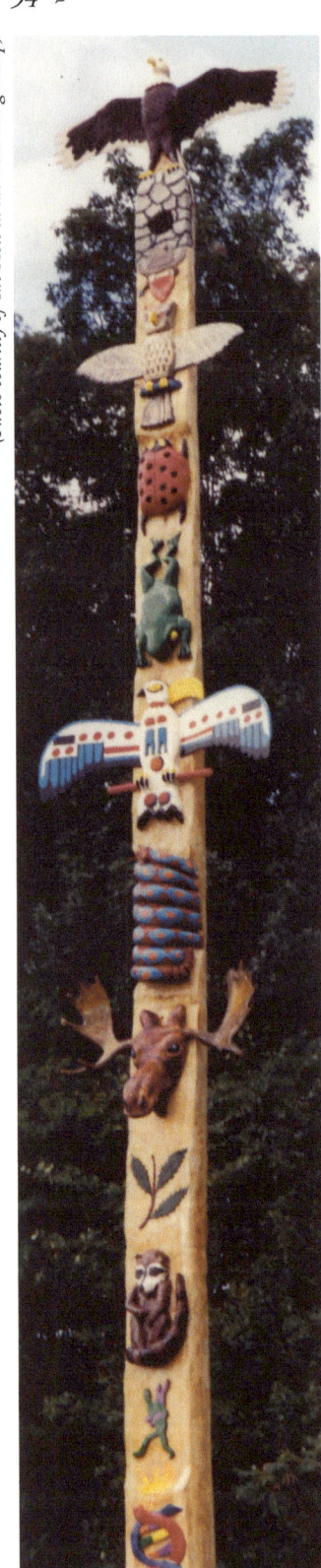

(Photo courtesy of The Hole in the Wall Gang Camp)

VIGILANCE

The Legend of VIGILANCE, 1994

*The EAGLE, soaring above pain and hardship,
and the children gather strength from their firm grip on
THE HOLE IN THE WALL GANG CAMP.*

*Like the OWL, children at Camp gain a special wisdom of themselves
and of their future.*

*The LADYBUG reminds the campers that although they have had misfortunes,
they will have their share of good luck.*

*The FROG, a Native American symbol of water.
At Camp the waters are tears of both joy and sadness.*

*The THUNDERBIRD, messenger between the Earth and Heavens,
symbolizes the special communication among the children because
of their shared experiences at Camp, communication that continues
long after the summer.*

*The coiled SNAKE, symbol of the paradox of the dangers and healing
of treatment.*

The GREAT NEWMOOSE, who made Camp happen.

*The AMERICAN CHESTNUT TREE, a symbol of courage and determination.
Cut to its rootstalk a century ago by a deadly blight,
it still sends green branches into the skies of Camp, again and again
and again.*

*The RACCOON, symbolic of capricious fate that can unexpectedly
and without reason
strike even the most innocent.*

*A COUNSELOR carrying a CAMPER, a symbol
of caring and closeness that is the most indelible Spirit of Camp.*

*A RISING SUN over the DOUBLE HELIX of DNA –
the human gene in the colors of the Camp Units.
Abnormal DNA causes many childhood cancers
as well as hemophilia, sickle cell anemia and thalassemia.
The hope and promise of the future are that these diseases,
through knowledge and more than a little luck, will be conquered
so The Hole in the Wall Gang Camp can become a bright memory.*

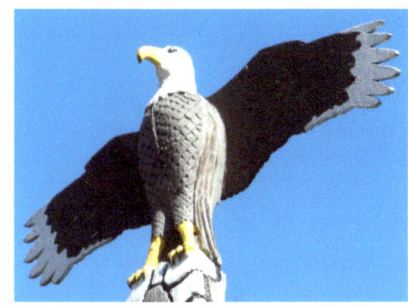
Noble 1994 eagle

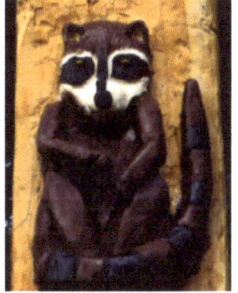
Mischievous raccoon

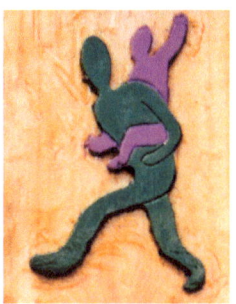
Counselor and camper

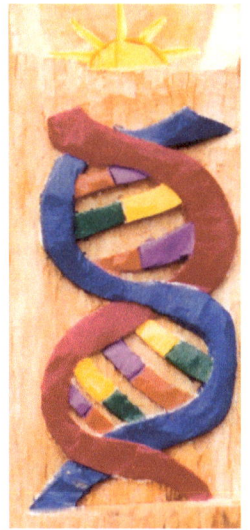
DNA, the double helix

In response to my request for a moderate-sized cedar in 1993, Paul ordered three huge, 75-foot, 100-year-old freshly cut white pine logs that were delivered from Maine in the spring of 1994. All three were turned into totem poles (1994, 1996, and 1998).

An eagle, nobly representing freedom and strength, is again a fitting symbol to place at the totem pole top, as it was in 1988. Camp gives children the strength and freedom of the eagle.

Below the recurring Little Bandit and owl totems is the good luck symbol—my second ladybug, a helpful insect that is fun to carve and paint.

As in the 1991 pole, the frog below the ladybug represents the water of Pearson Pond and the tears of joy and sorrow. I used bright marbles for the eyes of this one. I carved a second snake (the first one was on the 1992 pole) to again display its symbol of both the danger of disease and treatments. Below the snake is Paul NewMoose, with real moose antlers that were found in nearby woods, and then another chestnut tree totem.

Like so many of our campers, the raccoon is mischievous and playful. Despite their innocence, children and raccoons can be struck by capricious fate or bad luck, as Paul recognized. At THITWGC, we provide children with opportunities to counteract the capriciousness of disease and bad luck, and the raccoon totem acknowledges this. In some Native American folk tales, the raccoon plays a trickster that outsmarts other animals. I liken the raccoon, with the "mask" effect of dark coloring around the eyes, to the "Little Bandit." Along with the children, they are at Camp to have fun and maybe outsmart disease.

The next totem shows both the physical and emotional bond between counselors and campers. Although golf carts are available when needed, counselors often carry campers who need extra help with mobility off the beaten path. Children, tired from disease, weak from chemotherapy, or disabled from cancer surgery (particularly those with brain cancer), often need assistance.

Next, medical research on DNA, the double helix, shows bright promise under the sun for treating, curing, and perhaps preventing some of the diseases of the campers. Through research, we are constantly learning more about the cancers and blood diseases that afflict our children.

VIGILANCE was originally placed near the Camp entrance. Because that low-lying area was too boggy, it was moved in 2007 from the Camp entrance to stand beside the Infirmary. In 2015, it was moved into the Dining Hall to preserve it.

CHAPTER 11 ~ Beyond Just a Camp Doc

The Legend of OLYMPICS, 1996

*The HOT AIR BALLOON, with Paul Newman in the basket below,
each summer lifts the children's spirits high,
but like their hopes, always remain tightly tethered to Camp.*

The SQUIRREL shaking his bushy tail to the cadence of the campers' songs.

*The RAINBOW with the five colors of the Camp Units,
arching high above the TEPEE and CAMPFIRE.*

*The THUNDERBIRD, enduring symbol of the special communications
with other campers and the Camp Family long after summer is over.*

The CADUCEUS is the healing of Camp.

*The HORSE that carries the children over the trails of Camp –
and also the outrageous WONKY the WONDER HORSE of the Theater.*

*The FLAMINGO, fantastic creature of Fidget the Clown
that embodies the artistry and imagination of Camp.*

*In the blue waters of the Pond swims the elusive WEE-PEE,
the great fish that no one has seen, but every camper wants to catch.*

*The COMPASS AND SUNDIAL, guiding the Camp and campers in the
right direction through the day.*

*The LITTLE BANDIT representing the campers and the HOLE IN
THE WALL.*

*The SPIDER, inspired by Sara Johnson, Sue's daughter,
who scribbled a black blob on the bottom of the log that was easily converted
to a SPIDER.*

*The OLYMPIC LOGO, five rings in the colors of the Camp Units,
acknowledges that the Flame of the 1996 Olympic Games
passed directly by Camp on its way to Atlanta.*

(Photo courtesy of The Hole in the Wall Gang Camp)

OLYMPICS

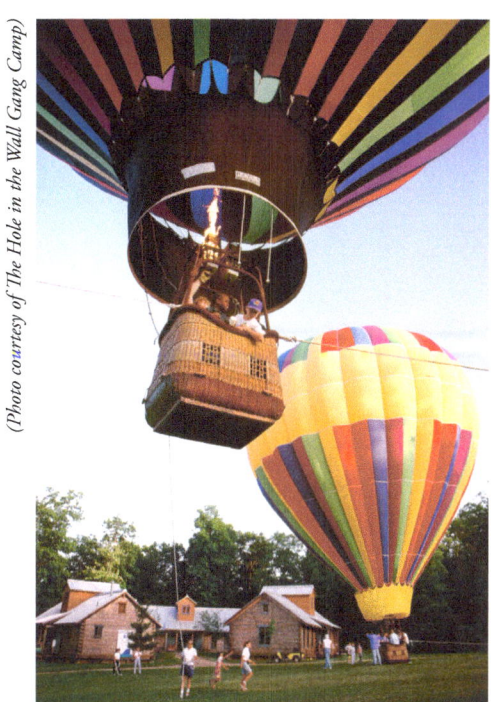
(Photo courtesy of The Hole in the Wall Gang Camp)

Hot air balloons visited Camp

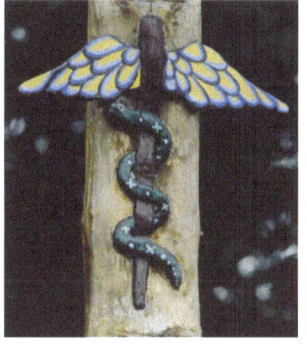

Caduceus, symbol of healing

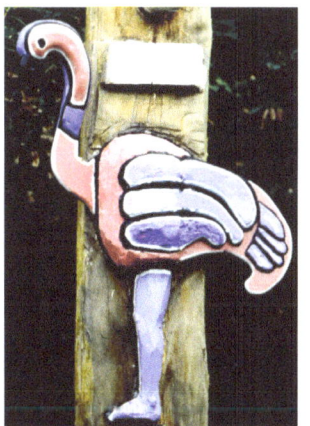

For Fidget and Flora

Before the 1996 Olympic Games happened in Atlanta, the Olympic torch was carried directly past Camp's entrance on its way across the country. Because of this, I named the 1996 totem pole OLYMPICS, and it tells stories about Camp activities and people.

The top totem was inspired by a volunteer hot air balloon group from Rhode Island that visited Camp to give children tethered rides in the balloons. Paul enjoyed going up in the balloons, and it is his figure seen in the basket waving down to Camp. The balloon appears to rise up into the sky.

The squirrel, often seen at Camp with its big bushy tail, is on the pole to represent after-dinner fun and dancing in the Dining Hall.

Beautiful rainbows are often seen over Pearson Pond and above Camp. I thought it fitting to place one on a pole and show the Unit colors as well. Below the rainbow is a tepee along with a campfire. There is something magical about gathering around a campfire under the dark, starry night with special friends.

Below the campfire, I carved a caduceus, originated long ago in Greece as a sign of medical healing. The snakes carved on earlier poles are part of the caduceus symbol, which likely has a biblical origin, Matthew 10:16: "Be ye therefore wise as serpents and harmless as doves." THITWGC can be an inspirational place of healing. It is fitting to have two of my symbols—the caduceus and Wonky the Wonder Horse—together on a totem pole. Underneath Wonky is a flamingo in honor of Fidget the Clown, who often dressed up in tandem with Flora the Flamingo.

The fish on this pole is the second representation of Wee-Pee, and I carved him again because of the popularity of fishing. The Wee-Pee legend is perpetuated year after year during fishing ventures, either from the dock or from boats.

Below Wee-Pee on the pole, I had originally placed a model of a compass and sundial made with laminated wood. It was a symbol about both THITWGC and our campers "going in the right direction." Unfortunately, it fell apart the first time it got wet in the rain. To replace it, I carved a hat and ukulele-sized octave guitar totem representing the props of Noodle the Clown.

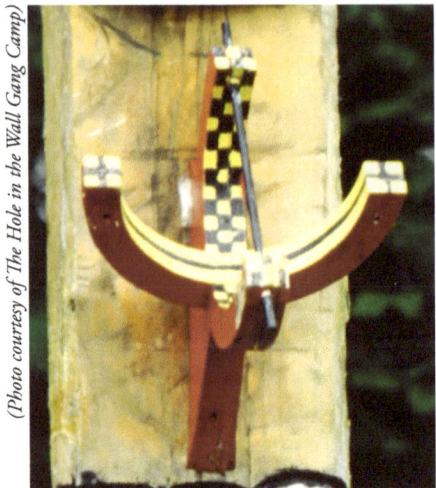
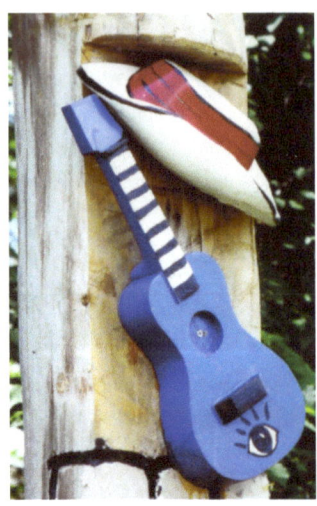
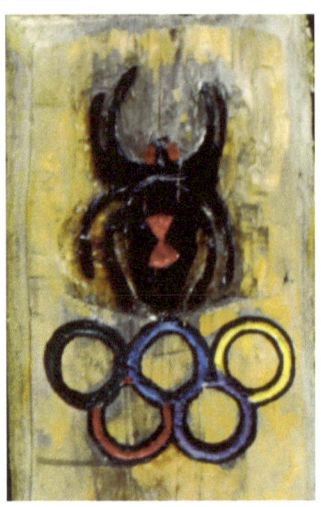

The original compass and sundial

Noodle's totem replaced the compass and sundial

Black-widow spider and Olympic rings

(Photo courtesy of The Hole in the Wall Gang Camp)

Next comes the hole in the wall, followed by a black-widow spider. Sara, the daughter of Sue Johnson, wanted to contribute. I gave her a black marker, which she used to scribble a black blob on the log that I easily converted into a spider.

At the bottom is the Olympic logo in the five colors of the Camp Units. In the summer of 1996 prior to the Olympic Games in Atlanta, the Olympic torch passed by the entrance to Camp on Route 44 on its way across the country. The counselors and campers during that session were gathered at the side of the road to cheer the runner with the flaming torch. But instead of a runner, a fast-moving motorbike whizzed by so rapidly that most of the children missed seeing the torch. Counselor Dorcas dashed back to the nearby Maintenance building, quickly fashioned a torch, and lit it with a flame. She ran back to Route 44 and jogged past the cheering campers with torch in hand in an appropriate reenactment.

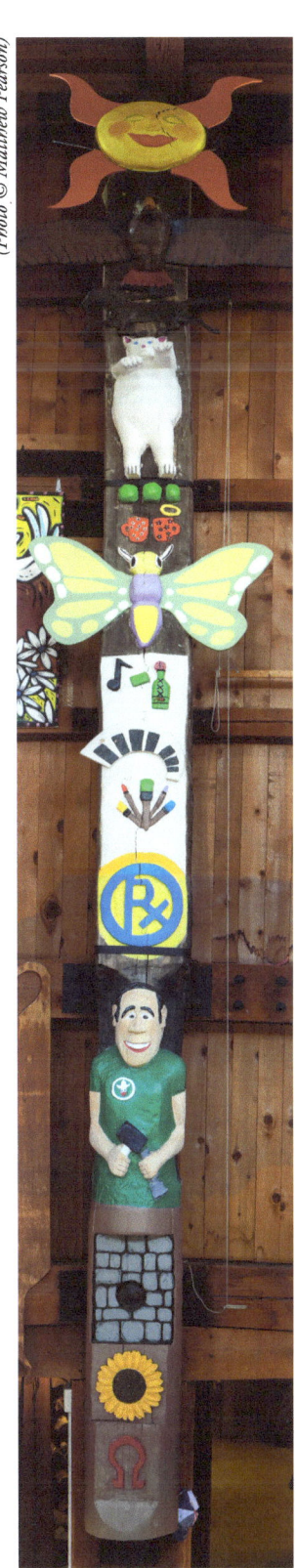

OMEGA

The Legend of OMEGA, 1998
--My tribute to ten years, 1988 – 1998, and to some of the people who made them memorable for me

The bright SUN, reflecting the beauty and warmth still radiating over Camp from some of the female campers and women leaders who have left us, including Annie, Alice and Sue L.

The RED-TAILED HAWK that flies over Camp and embodies the spirits of some of our male campers, including Mike.

The HORSE, for my favorite equestrienne, Jennifer, and the Horse Barn Crew, who bring joy to the children and to me.

The POLAR BEAR and COFFEE CUPS, for my early morning coffees on the porch of the Wood Shop with Dan, Chris, Joey, and Father Dominick.

The GREEN PEAS, in tribute to the cooking skills of Charlotte and other cooks who fed our bodies, as Camp fed our souls.

The LIGHTNING BUG, whose gentle glow lights the Camp paths in the summer evenings, like the sparkles in the children's eyes.

The KEYBOARD and MUSICAL NOTE, symbolizing the musical magic of Leo, as well as the GREEN CARD that he worked so long to get and his HOT SAUCES that livened the Dining Hall for some.

The PAINT BRUSHES, in the colors of the Camp Units, as my tribute and thanks to my artists and totem pole painters, especially Sherry and Anne.

Rx, the healing symbol of the Infirmary, Sue, and my nurses.

The TOTEM POLE CARVER (me) with my mallet and chisel helping to shape THE HOLE IN THE WALL GANG CAMP.

The SUNFLOWER, the official Camp flower.

OMEGA signifies my last Totem Pole.

At the top of this last totem pole, I carved a brilliant sun to represent some wonderful women who have passed away. Among them were Annie, Alice, and Sue L. Annie and Alice were on Camp's Board of Directors. Alice's husband, Calvin "Bud" Trillin, an author and frequent contributor to *The New Yorker* magazine, also came to Camp. He taught children how to slice a banana before peeling it by using a needle and thread. When the banana is then peeled, it is already sliced! He made it look like magic. Sue L. was a camper as a child and a counselor as a young adult.

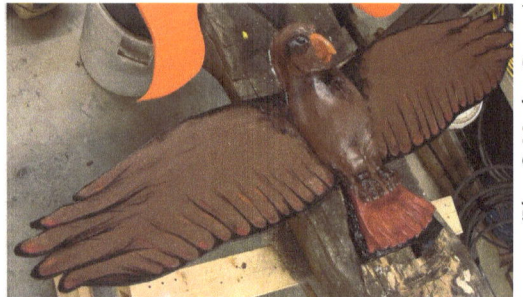

Red-tailed hawk, for Mike

The red-tailed hawk below the sun was inspired by Mike, one of my long-time thalassemia patients. He, too, was a camper and later a counselor. I carved this for Mike and others who have passed away. After Mike died, his mother said that she missed her son but knows that his spirit still flies over Camp as a red-tailed hawk.

Affixed on the pole is one of the metal horses decorating the walls of the Infirmary. This totem honors the well-behaved, gentle horses of the Horse Barn and Jen.

On most days, staff, volunteers, and campers could do some activities before breakfast. We called them Polar Bear Activities, and the polar bear on the pole symbolizes them. Father Dom, Cappy, Chris, Joey, and I had an informal "Polar Bear Club." We would meet before the Camp day started, to drink coffee (hence, the mugs on the pole) and talk on the porch of the Wood Shop. The yellow halo above one of the coffee mugs honors Father Dom.

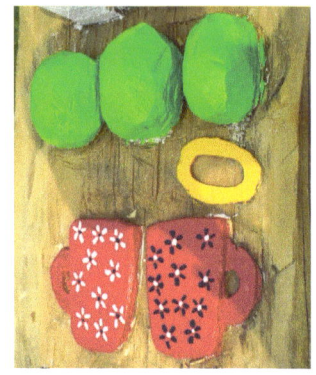

Charlotte's peas, Father Dom's halo, and our coffee mugs

The three green peas below the polar bear represent Charlotte, the tireless Head Cook for many years, and the general cooking and kitchen staff members. They provide nutritious and tasty food not only in the Dining Hall but also for special events, such as campouts in the tepees. There is an alternative explanation for the totems of the polar bear and peas that I attribute to some counselors, who circulated a joke about how Eskimos catch polar bears—they cut a hole in the ice and place three peas on the edge of the hole. When a polar bear comes along to "take a pea," they kick him in the "ice hole."

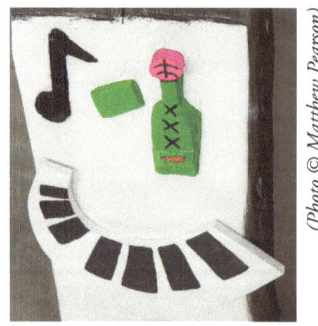

Leo's totem: musical note, green card, hot sauce, and keyboard

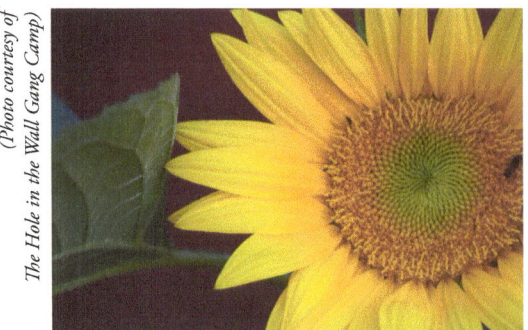

Flower of THITWGC

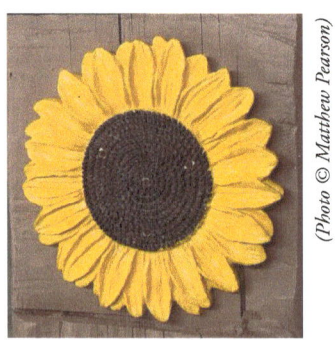

Sunflower on OMEGA

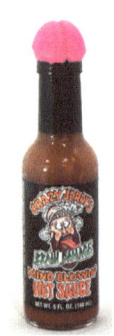

The real hot sauce

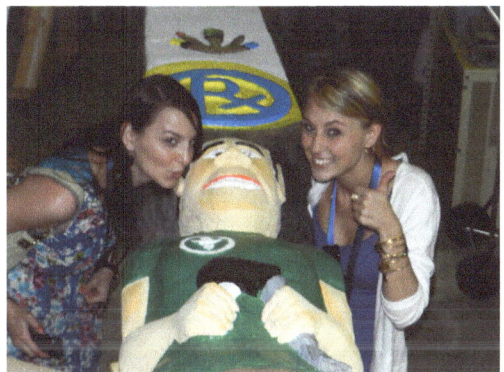 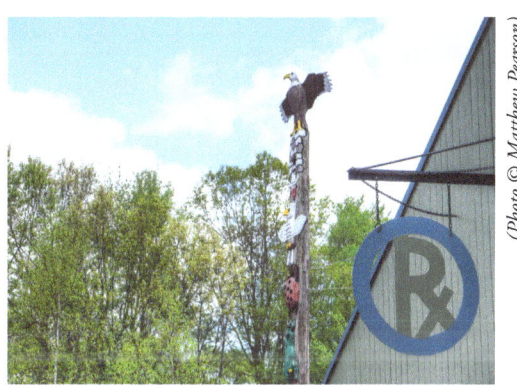

"Here's our Grampy!"   *Infirmary Rx sign, with VIGILANCE in the background*

    Below the mugs, I carved a lightning bug. Also known as fireflies, these bugs come out in the evening during the early part of the summer to intermittently light up their abdomens in a magical glow. The little flashing bugs remind me of the sparkles of happiness that light up in the eyes of campers.

    Underneath the lightning bug is a complex totem for Leo, the super-talented Russian musician who provided joy through music to all. At the time I carved this pole, Leo was facing a challenge to secure his green card, which he needed to continue working in the U.S. I traveled to Boston to testify on his behalf at the judicial hearing, part of the green card application process. I introduced myself to the judge, and he exclaimed, "Oh, hell! I thought Paul Newman would come!" Leo eventually received a green card and finally became a naturalized United States citizen in February of 2014. He continues to work in this country as a musician. When my pediatrician son Stephen first volunteered at Camp, he discovered that Leo shared his love of hot sauce. When he came to a session, Stephen would order a selection of his preferred sauces and store them in the kitchen. At each meal, he would bring the sauces to the table to share with Leo and others who dared to use them. One of their favorites had a plastic pink brain attached to the lid—which is depicted on the totem pole.

    My painters Anne and Sherry are represented as the paintbrushes in the colors of the units. Below the paintbrushes is the Rx symbol, almost identical to the metal sign hanging outside of the Infirmary. Rx means "prescription." Originally from the Latin word "recipere," which means "to take," Rx is the way a medical provider instructs a patient to take medicine or follow medical orders. The medical and nursing support at the Infirmary ensures that the Camp experience is safe for the children while remaining unobtrusive, as Paul had intended.

    As I was carving this last totem pole, Paul marked off about four feet in the lower section of the log. He instructed me to leave this space for him. After I finished the rest of the pole, Paul commissioned local artist Rick Champagne to place my image in the unfinished section. He depicted me carving myself into the totem pole. My family has always enjoyed that section of the pole, as shown in the photo with my granddaughters Paloma and Sarah.

    Just below the hole in the wall is a bright yellow sunflower. Because sunflowers are so plentiful around Camp, I carved one on a pole for the second time and proclaimed them as the official flower of THITWGC.

CHAPTER 11 ~ Beyond Just a Camp Doc

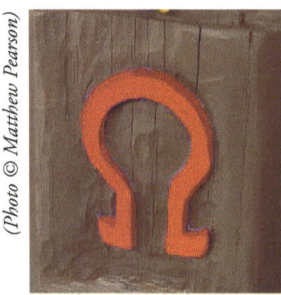

(Photo © Matthew Pearson)

Omega

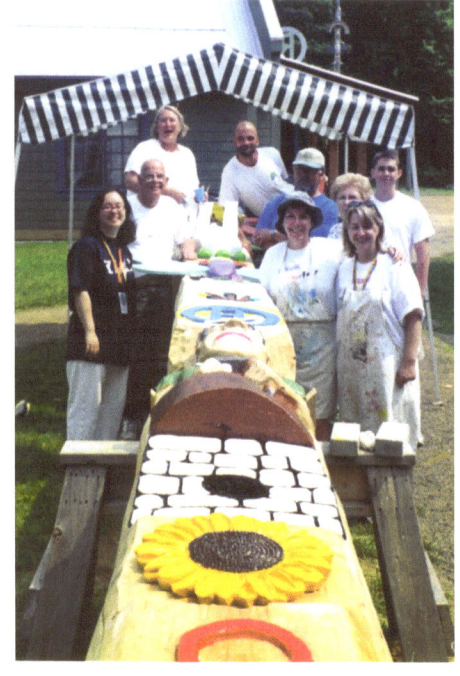

OMEGA painters—starting on the left and going around the pole: A Yale medical school volunteer, me, Sherry, Cappy, my pediatrician son Stephen, my grandson Daniel, Anne, my daughter-in-law Mary Lou, and a visiting pediatrician.

Omega, the last of the 24 letters of the Greek alphabet, is often used to indicate the last or an end of a series. This last totem symbolizes the conclusion of my creation of totem poles at THITWGC. It is similar in shape to a horseshoe, which is also a symbol of good luck.

Although Anne and Sherry were the primary totem pole painters, others pitched in when their time permitted. Three of my family members besides Anne—Stephen, Mary Lou, and Daniel—helped paint OMEGA. I had several other members of my family involved in Camp over the years. However, I also feel that the people at Camp became part of my extended family. My role as pediatric hematologist/oncologist in the Infirmary helped make Camp safe for the children, but being a pole carver and creating totems symbolic of the spirit and magic of THITWGC brought me closer to my extended Camp family.

Totem Pole Repair

Over the years, the totem poles have been damaged by nature—the harsh and snowy winter weather of Ashford, termites, woodpeckers, and mice. As already mentioned, we lost the pole called HOPE and part of CREATION. When I visited Alaska in 2011, a Native American totem pole carver informed me that Pacific Northwest poles also deteriorate.

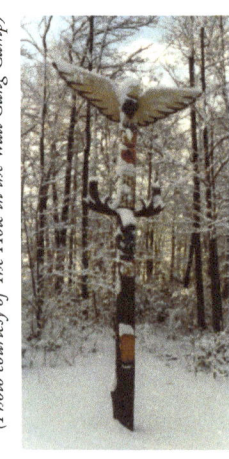

(Photo courtesy of The Hole in the Wall Gang Camp)

PROMISE weathering during a snowy winter

We have periodically used scaffolding and cherry pickers to repaint and repair some of the poles while they remained outdoors. On OLYMPICS, the hot air balloon lost a significant piece of wood, and Paul's hands went missing. My totem on OMEGA lost its glasses and chunks of the skin paint. VIGILANCE showed evidence that mice were eating the antlers of Paul NewMoose because their points were disappearing. In the wild, mice eat the shed antlers for their calcium content. THITWGC took steps to save the existing totem poles by moving them into the Dining Hall. PROMISE and CREATION were the first poles to be hung high on the walls. The repaired remains of SPIRIT were initially placed near the exit door. These three are smaller than the later poles.

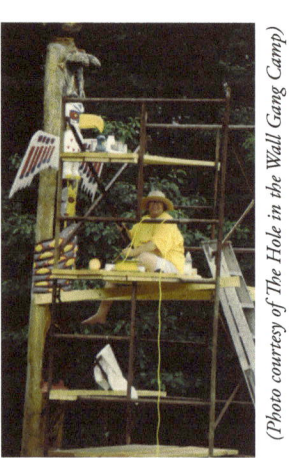

(Photo courtesy of The Hole in the Wall Gang Camp)

Sherry on scaffolding, repainting FULFILLMENT

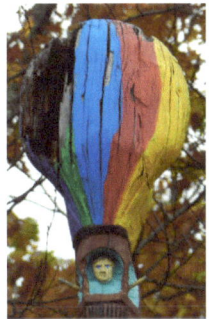
The balloon is disintegrating, and Paul's hands are gone

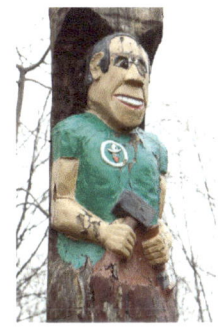
I am weather-worn, and I lost my glasses

In the spring of 2013, a plan was developed to move the rest of my totem poles indoors to preserve them so that they might continue to delight the children of the Hole in the Wall Gang Camp in the future. FULFILLMENT, WHIMSY, and OMEGA were moved to a maintenance building to be refurbished. Staff member Rebecca Patenaude enlisted the help of Camp alumni to repaint them. An engineering firm developed plans for the indoor placement of these large, heavy poles. They designed iron brackets sturdy enough to hold the poles and elevate them in order to maintain adequate Dining Hall floor space. In March of 2014, the three poles were set onto their elevated brackets using a winch and crane. OMEGA was reported to weigh 800 pounds. Now secure and safe indoors, they reach the top of the Dining Hall's towering round ceiling. OLYMPICS and VIGILANCE were refurbished and moved into the Dining Hall in the spring of 2015.

What luck that the remaining eight totem poles are now mounted on the walls of the circular Dining Hall! It is as if Tom Beeby had designed the building to perfectly accommodate them.

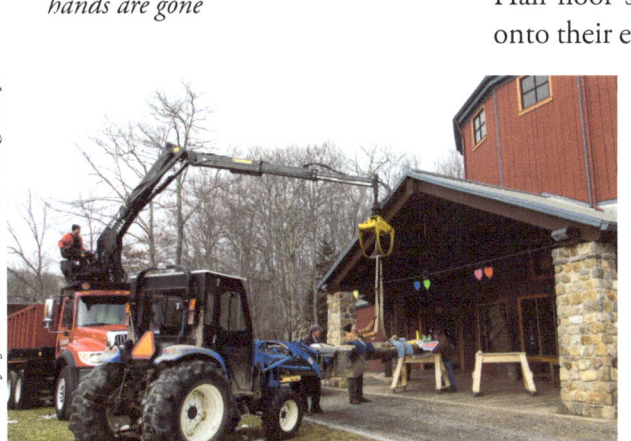
(Photo courtesy of The Hole in the Wall Gang Camp)
Transferring the repainted FULFILLMENT into the Dining Hall in 2014

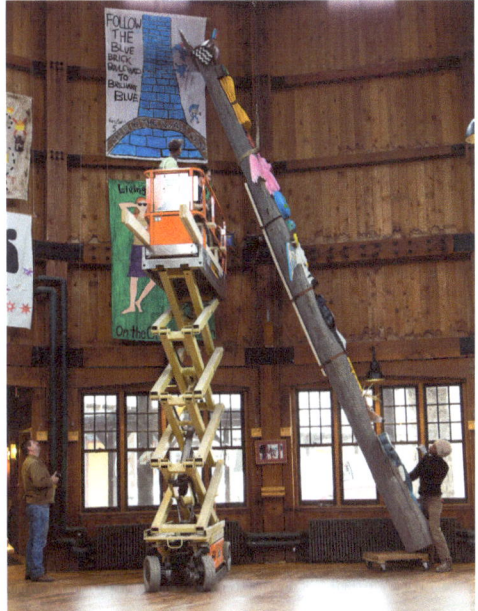
Lifting repainted WHIMSY to a vertical position indoors

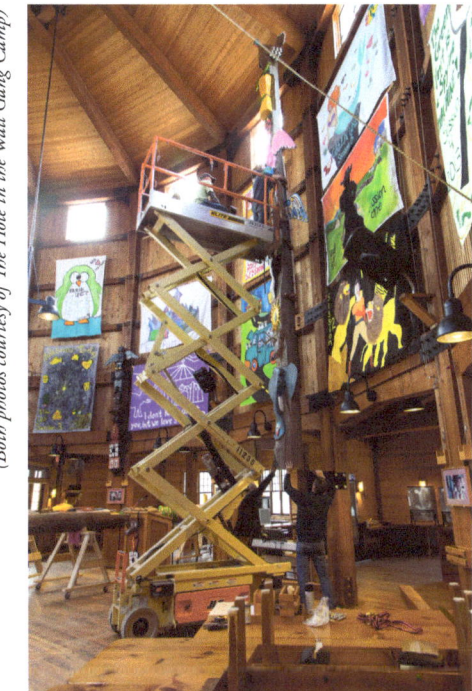
(Both photos courtesy of The Hole in the Wall Gang Camp)
Setting WHIMSY on its brackets

Totem Pole Paraphernalia

Over the years, I have acquired a number of treasured mementos related to the totem poles that bring back memories about THITWGC. Anne has skillfully and lovingly painted a series of miniature wood replicas that I carved of the first seven poles. She did it with the same patience she had while painting the poles at Camp. We display them in our living room.
(All miniature pole photos © Matthew Pearson)

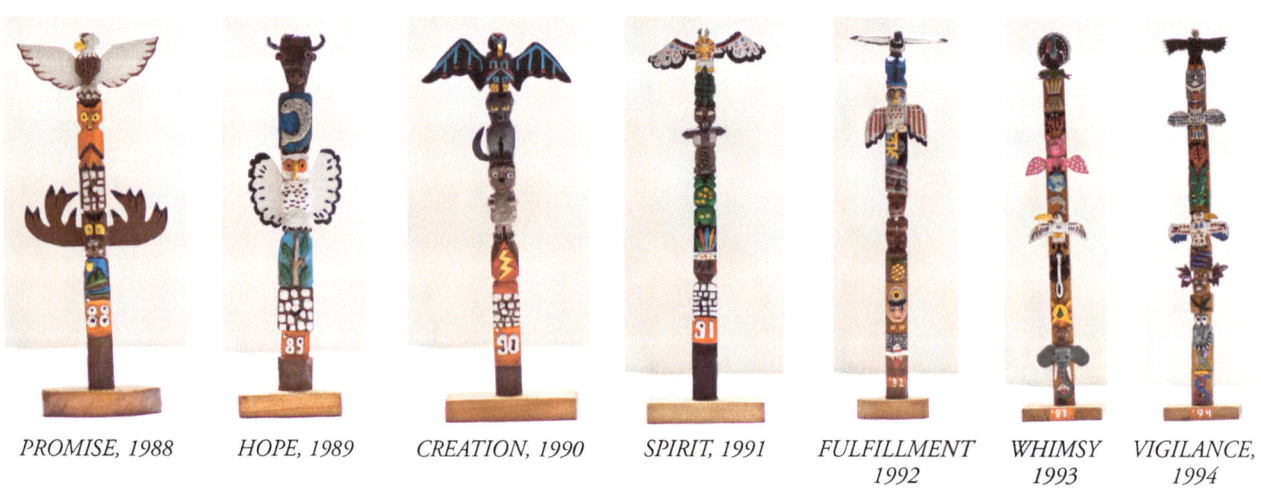

PROMISE, 1988   *HOPE, 1989*   *CREATION, 1990*   *SPIRIT, 1991*   *FULFILLMENT 1992*   *WHIMSY 1993*   *VIGILANCE, 1994*

My old high school friend, artist Armand Sindoni, sketched the 1988 and 1989 poles for use on my holiday cards. Starting in 1990, my son David did the sketches. These cards allowed me to share my Camp experiences with friends and family each year.

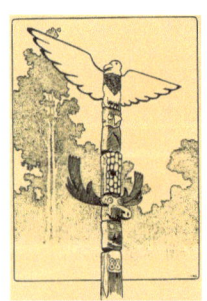 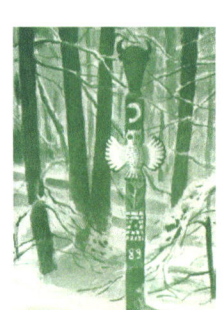 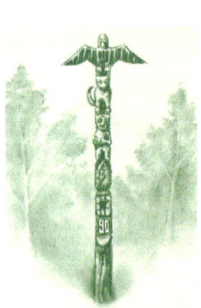 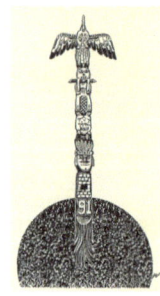 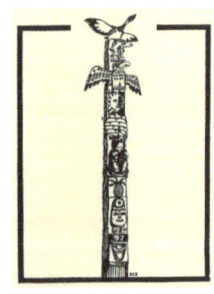

PROMISE, 1988   *HOPE, 1989*   *CREATION, 1990*   *SPIRIT, 1991*   *FULFILLMENT, 1992*

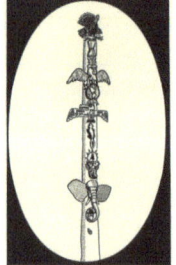 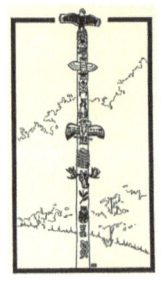 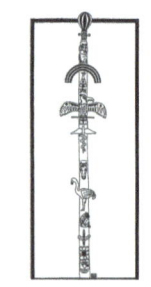 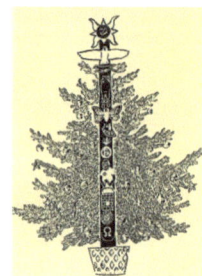

WHIMSY, 1993   *VIGILANCE, 1994*   *OLYMPICS, 1996*   *OMEGA, 1998*

Mary Lou created nine cloth totem pole replicas that grace our home, causing a "vertical effect," according to Anne. I can reminisce at home by gazing at these Christmas gifts from her. At my request, Mary Lou duplicated a couple of them for Paul. He hung the PROMISE replica in the poolroom of his and Joanne's cabin at Camp.

After the cloth totem poles that Mary Lou sent me as Christmas presents in 1988 and 1989, each year I would send her close-up photographs of my newest totem pole upon its completion, with the hope that she would create another wall hanging. When Mary Lou's packages arrived at our home during the holiday seasons, I could not resist opening them immediately. In addition to the cloth totem poles, she also made some shirts with hand-embroidered totem poles on them for Paul, Anne, and me.

May Camp's spirit and magic, expressed in my totem poles, help sustain and inspire campers, counselors, families, and friends as long as THITWGC is needed.

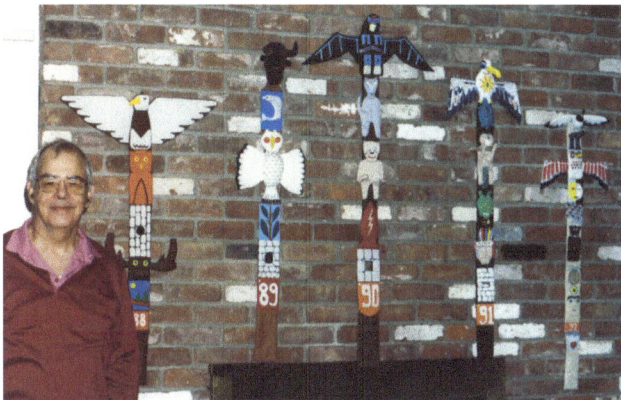

With the first five cloth totem pole replicas in my living room

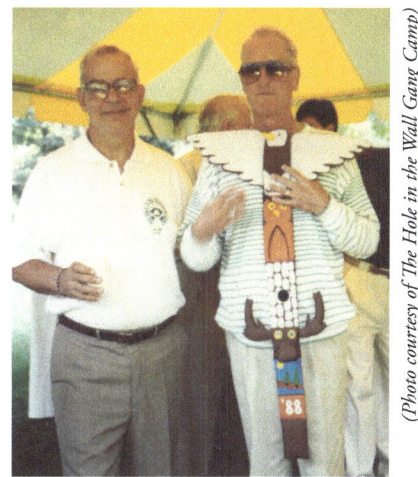

Presenting a cloth PROMISE to Paul, 1991

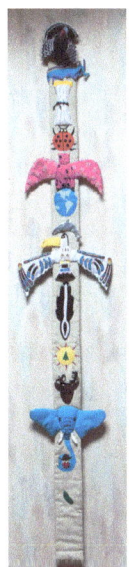
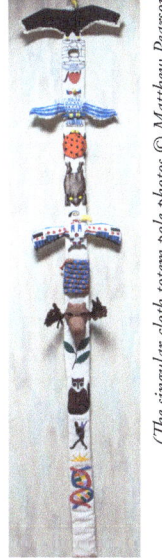
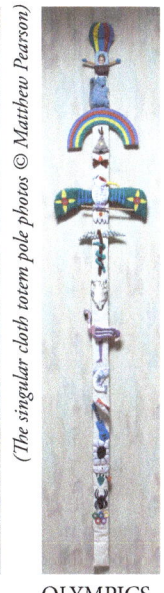
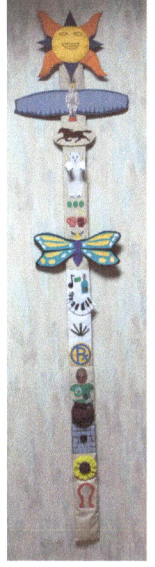

WHIMSY   VIGILANCE   OLYMPICS   OMEGA

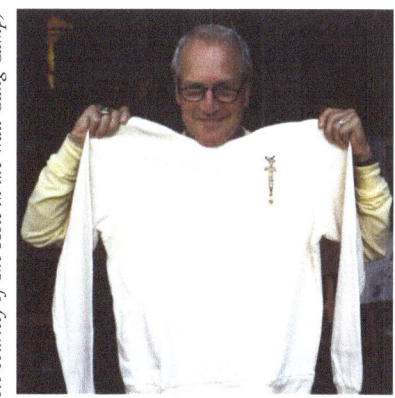

Paul with his VIGILANCE shirt from Mary Lou

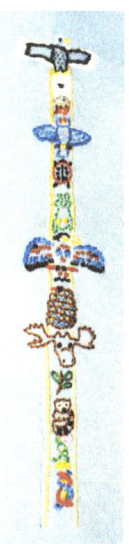

Close-up of Mary Lou's hand-embroidered VIGILANCE on a shirt

Honored by Paul

In the mid 1990s, Paul gave me a sterling silver totem pole that he designed and commissioned for casting by a New York City silversmith. Elements from the Camp poles are depicted, including an owl, the face of a person, a wingless thunderbird with a long beak, and a hole in the wall. At the base of the pole, he placed an engraved inscription to me: "To the Medicinal Magician with Considerable Affection and High Regard from Great Bull Newmoose."

Paul was often colorful and witty when paying someone a compliment. I was amused and flattered when he described my role at Camp: "What Jefferson, Madison, and Washington were to the original states, Howard Pearson is to the Hole in the Wall Gang Camp, plus a generous splash of Spencer Tracy and a hint of Houdini."

On the occasion of my becoming a Professor Emeritus at the Yale School of Medicine in 1999, there was a celebration at Camp. At the event, Paul said of me, "Like Caesar was to Rome, like Shakespeare was to theater, like John Donne was to poetry, like Marilyn Monroe was to Hollywood, Howard is to children." Unbeknown to me, Paul had commissioned a bronze bust of me that he presented during the occasion. At Yale, retiring physicians often have oil paintings of themselves commissioned for hanging in the medical school or hospital. I decided that my bronze bust could evoke "pedestal envy" in retiring professors, so I took it to Yale-New Haven Hospital in lieu of an oil portrait. It was on display for many years in a hallway of the pediatric area. It now resides in the Pearson Conference Room, where medical students and pediatric residents are known to rub the bust's head for good luck.

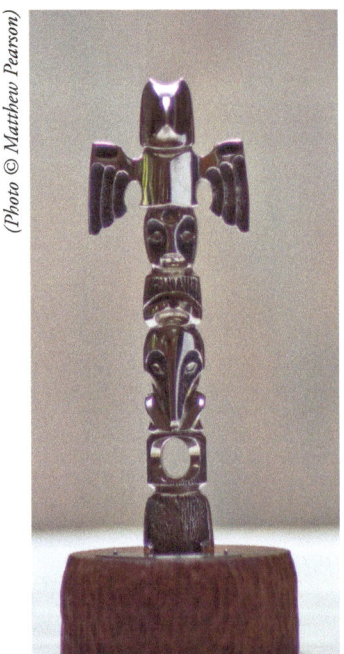

A gift from Paul—a sterling silver totem pole he designed and commissioned

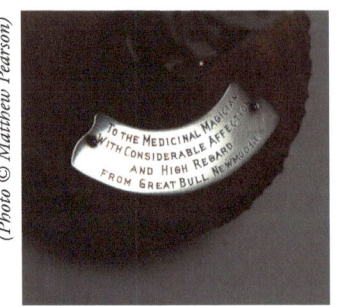

Inscription on the base of the silver pole

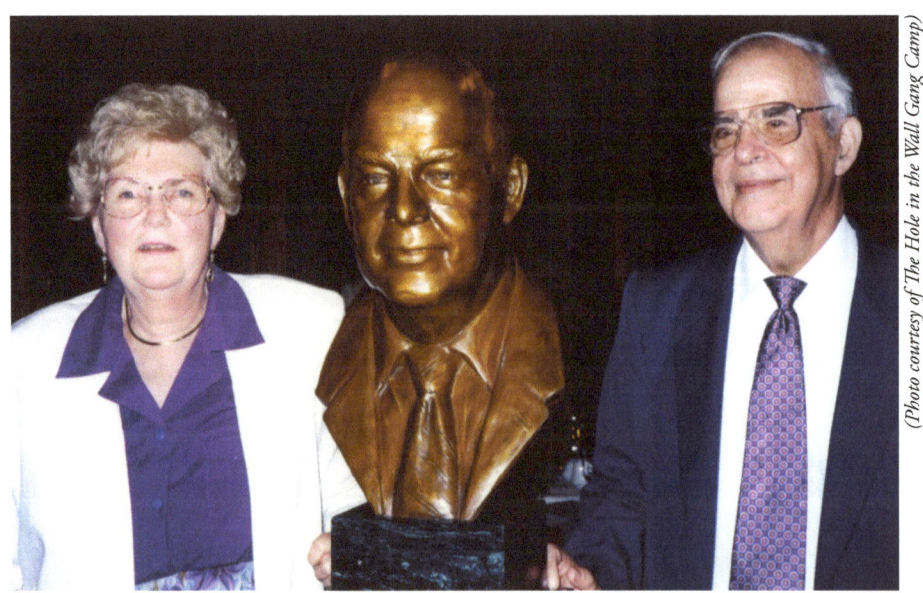

Bronze bust, commissioned by Paul and presented to me at Camp in 1999

Epilogue

Until I became involved with Paul Newman and his dream to have a camp for seriously ill children, I was a full-time pediatric hematologist/oncologist in the tertiary care hospital setting. At THITWGC, in addition to providing specialty care to the children, I served as their general pediatrician and as the physician for on-site staff. An occasional parent or outside doctor who did not know my background would sometimes approach me as if I were a general doctor at a camp for healthy children, but "Doc" at The Hole in the Wall Gang Camp is perhaps the proudest title I have ever had. Paul made it all possible with outstanding success. I honor him with this story from my perspective.

When I stepped down from the Board in 2014, Dr. Gary Kupfer, the current Chief of the Division of Pediatric Hematology/Oncology at the Yale School of Medicine and Yale-New Haven Hospital, was named to the Board at my suggestion. Gary had been a volunteer at Camp for several years and knows the needs. I strongly feel that the input of an influential and knowledgeable pediatric hematologist/oncologist at the Board level is critical to maintaining a high degree of safety and sensitivity to the medical needs of campers.

While I no longer have a formal position with THITWGC, I still visit when I can to feel once again the magic of the place. There is now a Founder's Garden next to the Dining Hall that acknowledges Camp's beginnings. Perhaps this book will preserve some of the history. My family tells me that I always look a few years younger when at Camp. But I looked old enough at the Camp's 2014 holiday party in the Dining Hall for a camper to gaze at me with wide eyes and ask, "Are you a Founder?" Surrounded by my totem poles in my favorite place on earth, I smiled and proudly replied, "YES!

Paul Newman's dream has been successfully fulfilled and sustained for over a quarter of a century. His leadership and persistence made it all happen. And I think he would heartily agree, if he were still physically with us today, that Camp continues to thrive, providing children with a place to "raise a little hell." His spirit remains at The Hole in the Wall Gang Camp.

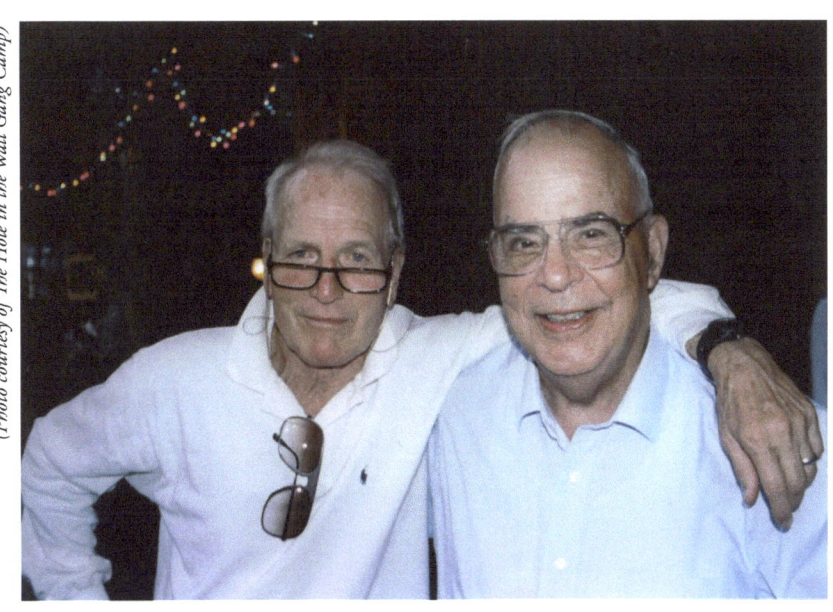

With Paul at Camp's 1989 holiday party

(Photo courtesy of The Hole in the Wall Gang Camp)

www.ingramcontent.com/pod-product-compliance
Lightning Source LLC
Chambersburg PA
CBHW042138290426
44110CB00002B/52